DIABETES

The Facts That Let You Regain Control of Your Life

Charles Kilo, MD
Joseph R. Williamson, MD
with
Dick Richmond

Illustrations by
Sherry L. Williamson

John Wiley & Sons, Inc.
New York • Chichester • Brisbane • Toronto • Singapore

Publisher: Stephen Kippur
Editor: David Sobel
Managing Editor: Ruth Greif
Production Service: Publications Development Company

Library of Congress Cataloging-in-Publication Data

Kilo, Charles.
Diabetes : the facts that let you regain control of your life.

1. Diabetes—Popular works. I. Williamson, J. R. (Joseph R.) II. Richmond, Dick. III. Title.
[DNLM: 1. Diabetes Mellitus—prevention & control—popular works. WK 850 K48d]
RC660.K495 1987 616.4'62 87-6136
ISBN 0-471-85801-3

20 19

We dedicate this book
to our families and
to the many generous supporters
and volunteers of the

Kilo Diabetes & Vascular Research Foundation

and to

Brother John

To the Reader

Despite the fact that diabetes mellitus is one of the most common and important health problems in the world today, it is still poorly understood and widely mistreated. Even among physicians, confusion and controversy surround the cause(s) and treatment of diabetes and its later complications. Because diabetes is such a complex, poorly understood disease, many physicians are uncomfortable, unwilling, or unable to answer many of the questions raised by diabetics and their families. It is not surprising, therefore, that people with diabetes often find it very difficult and frustrating to get help in understanding why they have diabetes; why they can't or shouldn't eat anything any time they want; what causes the acute, and the long-term complications of diabetes; and how to live with diabetes and delay or avoid these serious complications.

We are both physicians, but we approach diabetes from two different directions. One of us (C.K.) is actively involved in treating and caring for large numbers of patients with diabetes as well as in research. The other (J.R.W.) is primarily involved in laboratory research on the cause(s) of vascular complications of diabetes. We have worked together for the last 20 years on a variety of research studies on diabetic animals as well as with people with diabetes to understand the importance of blood glucose control and the role of heredity and other factors in the long-term complications of diabetes.

Our purpose in writing this book is to share with you some of the insights we have learned about diabetes. We begin in Part One by taking an in-depth look at what diabetes is and what is really going on in the body of a person with diabetes—the roles of heredity and environment, and how age, weight, and sex can determine the way diabetes may affect you.

Because the controversies over research and how to treat diabetic patients have often confused not only diabetics but also many physicians, we offer some straight talk about diabetes research—past, present, and future—in Part Two.

Part Three on treatment is included because our experience convinces us that every diabetic wants to know what to do and how to do it to better manage his or her disease and to insure long-term health. *Normalization* is the key word here and we give specifics on how this can be achieved and why it is so important to every diabetic.

Finally, our main goal is to help diabetics and their families live with diabetes and to avoid or delay the complications. To this end, we offer some suggestions on how to identify physicians and other healthcare professionals who can teach the diabetic how to manage the disease to achieve the best control possible for today and for the future.

CHARLES KILO, M.D., F.A.C.P.
JOSEPH R. WILLIAMSON, M.D.

Acknowledgments

We have many people to thank for their help in preparing this book and for their guidance and belief in our work over the years.

To our good friend and colleague, Dr. Paul Lacy, who brought us together over 20 years ago, we offer our deepest thanks for the direction he gave our careers and for his continued interest in our research. To our colleagues, laboratory personnel, and to the staffs at Washington University School of Medicine and the Kilo Diabetes & Vascular Research Foundation, our appreciation for their patience and assistance through many projects including this book.

A particular thanks to Jackie Dudley, R.N./Diabetes Educator and Jeanne Rogers, Executive Director of the Kilo Foundation, for their contributions. Jackie brought her expertise and experience to the chapters on diet and education. Jeanne skillfully coordinated the editing of numerous revisions of the manuscript which benefited greatly from her journalistic talents.

For the hours of typing, our thanks to Beverly Cantoni of the Kilo Foundation.

Of special note, we had the pleasure of again working with Dick Richmond, a good friend and fine journalist. With years of newspaper experience to his credit, he helped us shape our thoughts and direct our approach so together we could write a book that is scientifically accurate while being clear and easy to read.

Finally, a very personal thank you to all the special people—young and old—with diabetes we have come to know over the years. Through their example of courage and hope, we have learned much and we have grown stronger in our own resolve and dedication to finding the answers to diabetes.

Contents

Part One The Disease 1

1. Understanding What Has Gone Wrong 3

Why Me? 3
Once You Know the Facts 4
The Root of the Problem 5

2. The Hard Facts 7

The Role of the Pancreas 7
The Two Types of Diabetes 11
How the Body Uses and Stores Energy 12
The Very First Signs 16

3. The Many Faces of One Disease 19

Searching for a Cause 20
The Type II Diabetic 22
Other Factors 26
Secondary Diabetes 30
The Potential Diabetic 31

4. Living an Active, Healthier Life 33

Who Must Take Insulin? 34
Oral Agents 35

5. The Truth about the Consequences 41

Strengths and Weaknesses of Our Cardiovascular System 42
Symptoms of Vascular Damage 48
Bad Nerves 49
The Risk of Blindness 51
Muscle Starvation 52

6. Victims of Heredity and Environment 53

What the Figures Say 54
Obesity and Predisposition 55
Evidence from Human Genetics 57
Responding to the Environment 58

7. How We Get Fat . . . How We Get Thin 63

How Our Fat Cells Work 64
Regulators of Appetite and Metabolism 64
Changing Your Eating Habits 68

8. Diabetes in Women 71

Urinary and Vaginal Infections 72
Sexual Function 72
Diabetes and Pregnancy 73
Susceptibility to Heart Disease 78
Joys of Life 79

9. . . . And in Men 81

Sexual Function 81
Nerve Damage 82
Use of Penile Implants 83
Reproductive Concerns 85

Part Two The Research and the Controversies 87

10. What We Know So Far 89

The First Effective Diabetes Treatment 90
Insulin: Where We Get It 91
Measuring Our Reserves 93

11. Controversies about Diabetes 97

The Genetic Viewpoint 98
Locating the Source of Damage 99
The Case for High Blood Sugar 99
How We Entered the Fray 101
Patients Who Are Difficult to Control 104
New Studies 106
References 108

12. Another Setback 109

The Reaction 110
References 115

Part Three Treatment 117

13. Education: An Essential Ingredient 119

The First Concerns 120
The Diabetes Educator 121
The Juvenile Diabetic 125
Listening, Counseling, Managing 127

14. Normalization of Blood Glucose Levels: Diet, Exercise, and Medication 131

Adapting Diet to Existing Habits 132
Determining Insulin Dosage 134
The Importance of Self-Monitoring 138
Achieving Normalization without Sacrificing Variety 140
The Importance of Exercise 142
Oral Agents: Who Is a Candidate? 146
Breaking the Routine 148

15. Planning the Diet 149

Bread and Starch Exchanges 150
Meat Exchanges 153
Fat Exchanges 157
Milk Exchanges 158

Fruit Exchanges 159
Vegetable Exchanges 160
Knowing the Numbers 162
Cholesterol and Saturated Fat Content of Various Foods 164
Free Foods 167

16. Alleviating Stress 169

Adrenaline Goes to Work 169
Controlling Stress 171

17. The Newest Approaches 175

New Technology 176

18. Choosing a Doctor 183

The American Diabetes Association 183
The Juvenile Diabetes Foundation 184
Getting Leads 184

Appendix A Resources 187

Appendix B Suggested Reading and References 188

Appendix C Cookbooks for Diabetics 191

Index 193

PART ONE

The Disease

CHAPTER 1

Understanding What Has Gone Wrong

Why Me?

"Why me?' is the first question almost everyone asks when told he has a chronic, potentially life-threatening illness. In the case of diabetes—as with so many illnesses—the answer may be painfully elusive. Even we physicians are often at a loss to explain what is happening; we know how complicated this disease can be, and that we, unfortunately, cannot always predict the range of its consequences. But so much is known today about managing diabetes, we feel the prognosis is better than ever before.

Mistakenly, some people think that diabetes is a minor problem like a cold. Some think that diabetes will go away in a few weeks. Others refuse to accept that they have it at all. For many people, acceptance of the fact that they have diabetes occurs in stages similar to those in the grieving process when accepting the death of a loved one. Most people who have been diagnosed as having diabetes have far too little information about the disease to understand and cope with it properly. When the "grieving" stages of *disbelief* and *denial* have passed, patients want to know HOW to survive. This begins the *coping* process. It involves changing and adapting one's lifestyle to accommodate the demands of this chronic illness—diabetes. Living with diabetes becomes a matter of exerting control. Control over daily habits such as eating and exercising, and control over many other factors we will discuss in later chapters. For everyone, control starts with education and understanding what diabetes is and how it affects the body.

Once You Know the Facts

A great many people who have diabetes initially find it difficult to accept the diagnosis. The first thing a doctor needs to do is to explain exactly what diabetes is and to get the individual and his family to accept the facts. Diabetes means high blood sugar (glucose) due to an absolute or relative lack of insulin. In addition, it is important to know that diabetes is not one, but many diseases. We can categorize diabetics into two major groups:

- *Type I* (insulin-dependent) People who are *dependent* on insulin injections to live because they no longer have adequate insulin production. This form is the most serious and affects primarily children and young adults.
- *Type II* (non-insulin-dependent) This form of the disease almost always affects people over age 30. They usually do not require insulin injections and can often manage their disease by carefully following a diabetic diet or by also taking one of the many medications available today.

What is not easy to explain and understand is how high blood sugar disrupts just about everything else happening in the body and how it can produce very serious, long-term consequences.

Today, approximately 13 million Americans have diabetes. Most, nearly 90 percent, have Type II. Diabetes is a disease where both heredity and environment play a part. It is a disease for which there is no known cure. While frightening and often depressing, this knowledge helps to emphasize the importance of management—of control—in learning to live with diabetes.

People often have to deal with very strong emotional reactions when they first learn they have diabetes. It is, therefore, important to know that there are many specially-trained health professionals who understand how to help them cope with their feelings and bring their disease under control. Diabetics can learn how to plan meals, inject insulin, self-monitor their blood glucose, and so on. At first, these new routines feel like a burden and an intrusion. Eventually, they become second nature as does any new skill or changed behavior. Once the basics about diabetes are understood, people usually gain confidence and want to learn more in order to acquire the skills that will enable them to regain control of their lives. Diabetics can go hiking and camping, carry on a normal social schedule, travel where ever they want, eat at fast food restaurants, and still take care of themselves. In short, people discover that they can live with this disease called diabetes; it is just a matter of getting through that very difficult initial period of adjustment and then continuing to learn, and modify their behavior as required.

The Root of the Problem

Just what is this disease? How does it come about? What are its effects? The answers to these questions are many and complex. In the next chapters we will explain what we know about these and other questions—what insulin is, why it is so essential to life, and why controlling diabetes is so important to your future.

We begin by identifying the root physical cause of diabetes which is an absolute or relative lack of the hormone insulin. Without an adequate supply of this hormone, the body is unable to utilize food properly, store nutrients we eat, or transform them into energy. When we eat, our body goes to work to convert food into various useful substances, discarding everything wasteful. It is the job of insulin to see that the useful substances are put to the best use for our well-being—for building cells, for immediate expenditure as energy, or for storage for future energy expenditure.

The three main substances controlled by insulin are glucose, fatty acids, and amino acids. Glucose is a simple sugar (carbohydrate) that fuels our immediate energy needs (particularly those of the brain); fatty acids (fats) are also utilized as fuel, especially in the heart and muscle, and are the storage form for calories consumed in excess of those that are burned for immediate use; and amino acids are the building blocks of protein and, therefore, of muscle. As glucose and fatty acids are metabolized and transported through the bloodstream, insulin—sometimes directly, sometimes with the help of other chemicals, such as enzymes—directs them to their proper destination and facilitates their uptake by the cells which need them. Without insulin, glucose, in particular, accumulates in the blood, and those parts of the body that need it become "starved" or unable to function properly.

Fatty acids that are not captured and retained by the fat cells—with the help of insulin—are released into the blood, carried to the liver, and converted into low-density lipoproteins. These lipoproteins are the carriers of cholesterol, which, in excess, we know is a major risk factor for hardening of the arteries and heart disease. Knowing the importance of insulin is the first step to understanding diabetes. In the next chapter, we will look more closely at metabolism in general and the vital role insulin plays.

CHAPTER 2

The Hard Facts

The Role of the Pancreas

The pancreas is located in the abdomen and is essential to the body's processing of food for energy. It is an oblong organ located below and behind the stomach and about one-tenth the size of the liver (Figure 1). Scattered throughout the pancreas are isolated clusters of cells known as the Islets of Langerhans (named for their discoverer, Paul Langerhans, a nineteenth-century German physician). Within these islets are located the *beta cells,* which are responsible for manufacturing and secreting the hormone, insulin, into the blood. Insulin (among its other tasks) helps the liver regulate the body's metabolism of carbohydrates.

Also in the pancreas are the *alpha cells,* which manufacture the hormone glucagon. Because they are concerned with hormonal matters such as regulating the activities of specific cells and organs, the Islets of Langerhans (Figure 2) are collectively known as the *endocrine pancreas.* These islets account for only about 1 percent of the entire volume of the pancreas.* The rest of this

*There are small numbers of other endocrine cells also present in these islets.

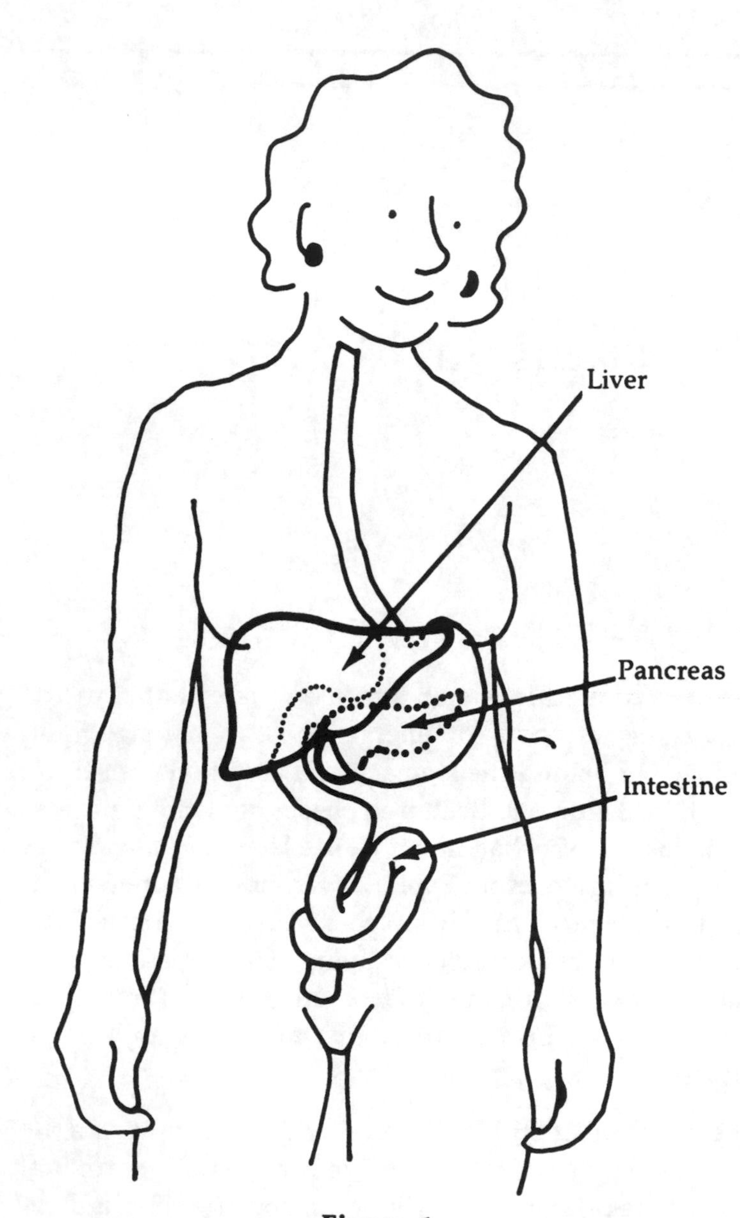

Figure 1

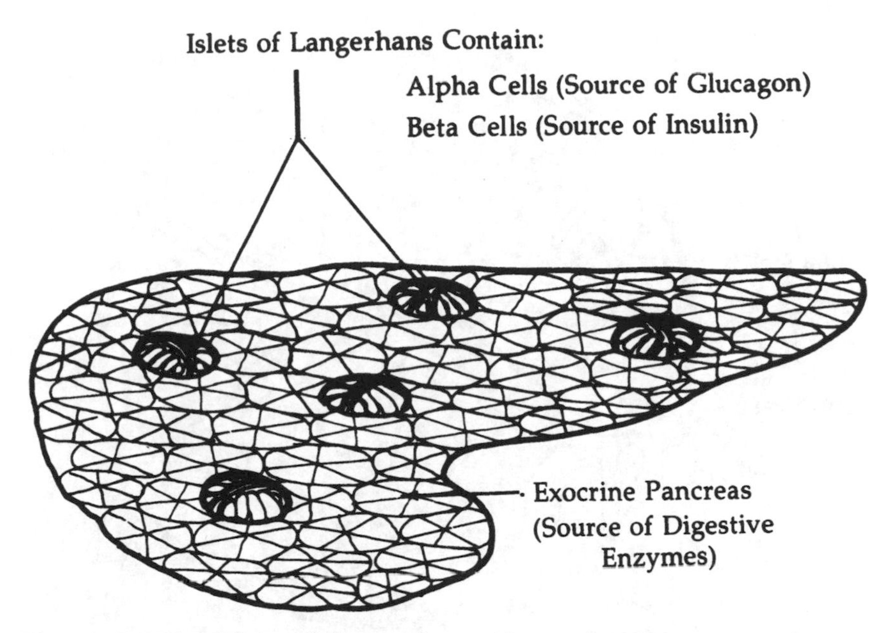

Figure 2 The Islets of Langerhans (the endocrine pancreas) are scattered throughout the pancreas.

organ, called the *exocrine pancreas,* makes digestive enzymes and secretes them into the small intestine. These enzymes break up food into smaller molecules, which are absorbed into the blood. Elevated blood levels of some of these, such as glucose and amino acids, trigger the beta cells to release their cache of insulin into the bloodstream, which distributes it to the rest of the body (Figure 3).

At least, that's how the system works in a person without diabetes. But in some diabetics, the insulin part of the cycle malfunctions. Because there is not enough effective insulin to promote uptake by the cells, glucose builds up in the bloodstream and circulates endlessly with nowhere to go. When the level gets too high, glucose spills over into the urine, taking with it the water and salts that are essential to survival.

A high level of glucose in the bloodstream is *the* most serious consequence of diabetes. Its potential for harming the entire

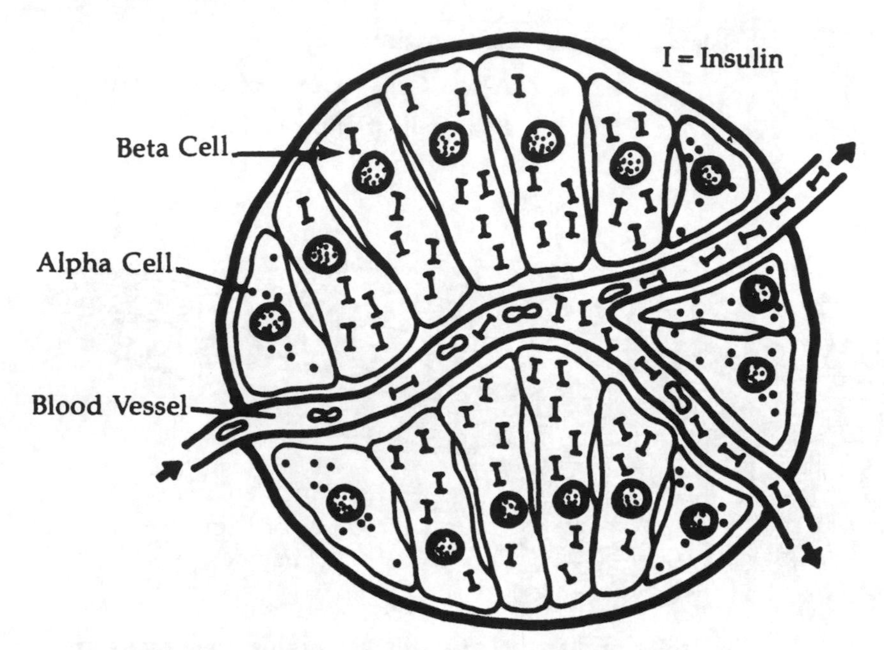

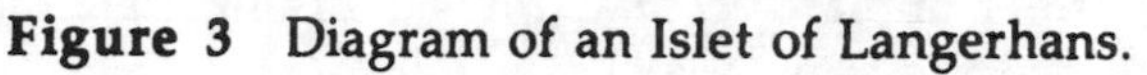

Figure 3 Diagram of an Islet of Langerhans.

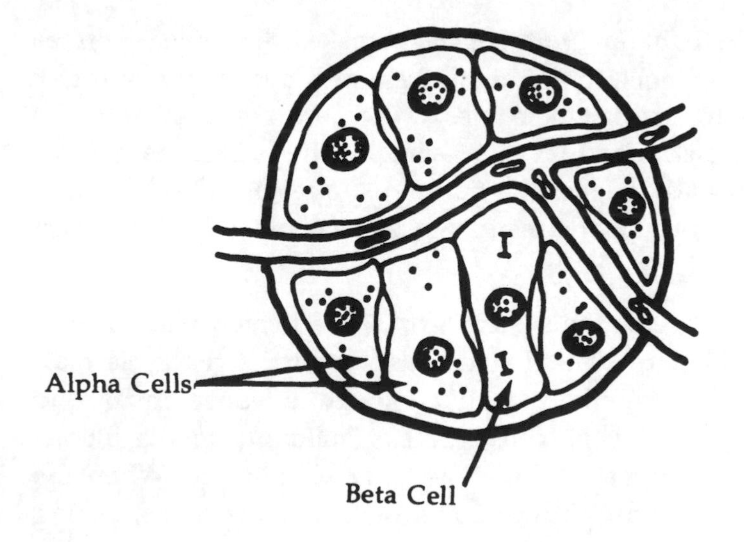

Figure 4 Islets of Type I diabetics are small and contain all or mostly alpha cells.

body should not be underestimated by patients or by physicians (as it has been until very recently).

The Two Types of Diabetes

Later on, we'll discuss at length the many specific effects diabetes has on our everyday lives, but it is essential to begin by differentiating between the different root causes of insulin deficiency.

Basically, there are two types of diabetes: Type I (insulin-dependent), once called Juvenile-onset diabetes, and Type II (non-insulin-dependent), formerly called Maturity-onset diabetes. Their symptoms can be similar, but their causes are quite different. In the Type I diabetic, almost all the beta cells have been destroyed so that daily injections of insulin become essential to life (Figure 4). In many Type II diabetics, these cells remain intact. The problem is not a failure of the beta cells to produce and release enough insulin, rather, the problem is the inability of the cells in the body that need it to respond. This is called *insulin resistance.* In other Type II diabetics, the beta cells may be able to produce sufficient amounts of insulin and store it but cannot release it. These variations are one reason diabetes is so complicated to explain and to treat.

In Type I diabetes, almost no insulin is being transported from the pancreas to the liver because there are few, if any, insulin-producing beta cells. In Type II diabetes, variable, but inadequate, amounts of insulin are transported to the liver. In both types of diabetes, the first serious problem affecting metabolism is that the liver does not function properly due to relative or absolute insulin deficiency. In Chapter 3 we'll discuss the two kinds of diabetes in greater detail, but for now we'll take a look at how metabolism normally works and the role the liver plays.

How the Body Uses and Stores Energy

All forms of life depend on metabolism for physical survival. Technically, the term metabolism refers to the chemical processes by which our bodies convert the foods we eat into cells and life-sustaining energy. Basically, we utilize (metabolize) foods in two ways: some of it is used to build and replenish cells throughout the body; the remainder fuels our activity and produces heat to maintain body temperature.

When we eat, all sorts of mechanisms are triggered. Within two or three hours after we eat, even a big meal, the food we have consumed has been broken down (digested) into forms that can be used by the body. These products of digestion are absorbed through cells that line the intestines and are taken by the blood to the liver (Figure 5). Elevated blood levels of glucose and amino acids from these products of digestion alert the beta cells in the pancreas to start releasing insulin into the blood, which ships this vital hormone directly to the liver, enabling the liver to remove glucose from the bloodstream. Normally, about two thirds of the sugar absorbed from a meal is taken up immediately by the liver. There, it is stored in the form of glycogen, which is later broken down into glucose and released into the bloodstream as needed. (Insulin also "signals" the liver to shut off sugar output when it has released enough for current demands.) The other third of that sugar is immediately available to the brain, muscle, and fat tissues, which may take it up directly from the bloodstream. The chief user of this glucose is the brain, which takes up some 60–70 percent of that immediate supply.

In diabetics, the liver no longer extracts as much glucose from the blood as it usually would; the shortage of insulin also means that other tissues, such as muscle and fat, cannot take their share of sugar from the bloodstream. The cumulative effect here is, obviously, a drastic build-up of glucose in the bloodstream and the virtual starvation of tissues that need insulin in order to take up and use glucose. On the other hand, the brain doesn't need insulin and it continues to take as much glucose as it needs.

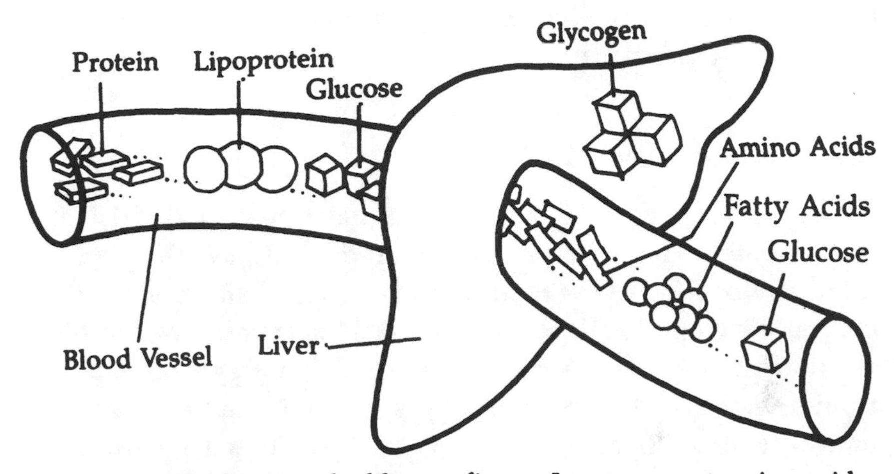

Figure 5 The liver works like a refinery. It can convert amino acids into proteins, fatty acids into lipoproteins and remove glucose from the blood, store it as glycogen, then release it again as glucose when needed.

Without an adequate supply of insulin, the liver is unable to take up enough blood sugar for storage while simultaneously being impelled to keep on producing it, since there is no insulin to shut it off. But once the liver has exhausted its store of glycogen, what can it use as a source for this runaway glucose production? Resorting to the body's alternative source of energy (ordinarily used only in times of starvation), the liver utilizes amino acids derived from muscles and converts *them* into glucose. Those amino acids are no longer available for re-use and maintenance of muscles and, as a consequence, the muscles atrophy (shrink).

The insulin's signal to the liver to stop making glucose is part of a critical biofeedback system. When the insulin level is high, it causes the blood sugar level to fall. If the blood sugar drops too low, then adrenaline, glucagon, and other hormones are released to bring the blood sugar level back up. (So actually, it is not only insulin, but insulin in concert with other hormones that regulate glucose levels throughout the body. Insulin, however, is the conductor.) When this biofeedback system is not functioning properly, the consequences can be tremendously destructive.

The Evolution of Metabolism

Our bodies have evolved over time to make maximum efficient use of whatever food we eat. Early man did not have the plentiful supply of food available now to Americans and the people of other developed nations. So in order to survive, it was to his advantage to be able to extract all potential energy from a paltry diet. Indeed, he spent most of his time getting food, facing times of feast or famine. His body "learned" to save extra energy gained in times of plenty so that it would be available during periods when food became scarce.

If you eat a big meal and absorb more energy-giving nutrients than you need at that moment, your body will store them for later use. For short-term energy needs, the liver's glycogen supply is readily available. Because of its bulkiness, glycogen is not efficient for long-term storage, but if, for instance, your brain begins to need more glucose, the liver can start breaking down glycogen and releasing it as glucose. Your brain is the primary user here, though other organs will take advantage of this supply, too. But most nutrients are stored in the form of fat. For the long term, fat is a very efficient storage form of energy. When you need it, it is released into the blood and carried to your muscle cells, which do the work for your entire body.

The reason fat is such an efficient way to store fuel is that it is compact, composed almost entirely of carbon and hydrogen. The air we breathe provides the oxygen necessary to burn the fat and produce energy.

Glucose, on the other hand, is a carbohydrate. Carbohydrates, which contain considerable oxygen as well as carbon and hydrogen, are a bulkier, heavier form of fuel as compared to fat.

Being water-soluble (fats are not), carbohydrates stored in the body tend to hold extra water, much like a sponge.

Generally, when we say that someone has a high or low rate of metabolism, we are referring to the rate at which the body burns fuel to produce energy. This rate varies widely from one individual to the next. There are differences in metabolic *efficiency* as well.

Even when we are at rest, we are metabolizing at a low rate. If we are working or exercising vigorously, we are metabolizing at a high rate. So the more physically active we are, the higher our overall metabolism, the more energy we use, and thus the more food we can eat without becoming fat. Insulin is a crucial factor in this cycle.

Insulin and Fat

There are two kinds of cells that burn sugar (glucose). One is easily penetrated by glucose without the aid of insulin. So the glucose level inside this type of cell is about the same as outside the cell. Examples of such tissues are the cells that make up our kidneys, brain, and blood vessels.

The second type of cell needs insulin in order to utilize sugar. Muscles and fat are made up of such cells. Insulin helps the sugar get into these cells so that they can burn it or store it for later use. Without insulin, the glucose simply cannot get through the cell walls (membranes), let alone be processed for energy. The exact mechanism by which insulin moves the glucose through the membranes is not yet fully understood.

Simply stated, then, insulin has the job of getting glucose into the fat cells and converting it into a form that can be stored. Insulin also regulates enzymes that break down blood lipids into fatty acids, which can cross the blood-vessel wall. After entering the fat cells, they are converted (again, with the aid of insulin) to a stable, storable form, so that they do not "leak" back into the blood.

As people get fat, their individual fat cells get bigger, and sometimes those cells seem to lose their ability to receive and hold onto insulin. Such cells are then less efficient at taking up glucose and burning it or converting it to fat for storage. In normal metabolism, as we've discussed, the sugar is taken up by the liver and by fat cells, and most of it is converted to fat for future use. Without insulin—or with the loss of an insulin-dependent cell's ability to *bind* insulin—this process becomes impossible, and glucose remains unused in the bloodstream, building up to dangerous levels and spilling over into the urine.

The Very First Signs

In many patients, sugar in the urine is the first signal that alerts a doctor to suspect diabetes. The measure for normal blood sugar is a fasting (before breakfast) level of 115 milligrams of sugar or less per 100 milliliters (1 deciliter, dl) of blood (115 mg/dl). After a big meal, it might rise to between 130 and 140 mg/dl (milligrams per deciliter). The level at which sugar will begin spilling into a person's urine is referred to as his *renal* (kidney) *threshold;* in the average person, that level falls between 170 and 180 mg/dl.

If all of us had the same renal threshold, it would be relatively simple for a doctor to diagnose diabetes from an analysis of sugar levels in urine. Unfortunately, different individuals have different thresholds. Consequently, a physician confronted with a urinalysis revealing the presence of sugar cannot be sure if it means that the patient has diabetes or simply that the patient has an unusually low renal threshold. And at the other end of the spectrum, some patients who *do* have diabetes, particularly those who have kidney disease as well, may not begin to show glucose in their urine until blood sugar reaches levels much higher than 170–180 mg/dl. This means that they could have an alarmingly high blood sugar level yet show falsely reassuring negative results on a urinalysis. So, unfortunately, the test for urine sugar is not always an accurate gauge of blood sugar levels. (This is the reason why the simple "strip test" which diabetics can perform at home to check urine for glucose cannot be relied on for great accuracy.) For diagnosis, the doctor must analyze and monitor the blood itself.*

Diabetes may also reveal itself through the condition known as *ketoacidosis.* In a person with an abnormally low insulin level, as is the case with Type I diabetics, excess fatty acids leak out of the fat cells into the blood because there isn't enough insulin to keep them properly stored. These fatty acids are carried to the liver and muscle tissues, which burn them as fuel. In the liver, the fatty acids are not completely burned up and the leftover substances, known as *ketones,* are produced at such a furious rate that they are released into the blood where they accumulate. Eventually, they spill over into the urine, and may even be breathed out of the lungs (in severe cases). This condition, which effectively poisons the whole body, cannot be ignored or serious consequences will result. (In the days before the discovery of insulin, this condition caused coma and death very quickly. And, even today, it can have the same results in a diabetic on insulin who does not properly manage the disease.)

**A Note about Glucose Tolerance Tests:* The use of this type of test to diagnose diabetes is no longer recommended. Still, such tests can be helpful in other ways when used properly. They will give the physician a clue as to how well a mild diabetic can metabolize a glucose load or large amount of insulin, which may be useful in developing the ideal diet for that individual. The poorer your ability to handle a glucose load, the more likely it is that your diabetes is worse than your fasting sugar level might indicate. If the fasting level is normal, and the two-hour blood sugar levels are higher than normal during a glucose tolerance test, then such an untreated person may be at high risk for developing overt diabetes unless he starts on a corrective diet and exercise program.

Such symptoms are but the tip of the iceberg when it comes to understanding diabetes and its potentially devastating effects on the body. The above discussion of metabolism gives a somewhat general picture of insulin's vital role in our survival, but the true complexity of its job will become increasingly clear as we examine specific cases of diabetes and the many issues—such as diet, exercise, and heredity—that doctors and patients must face.

CHAPTER 3

The Many Faces of One Disease

A nine-year-old boy, who had dropped in weight from 70 pounds to 57 pounds in a few weeks, was brought to his doctor for treatment. He had lost all that weight in spite of the fact that he was eating and drinking all the time, trying to satisfy a constant hunger and thirst. And he was forever going to the bathroom to urinate. He had even wet his bed—something he had not done since he was a baby.

Seven months earlier, the boy had had a routine physical examination. Because his doctor had so recently given him a clean bill of health, the parents were slow to realize that their son might have a serious illness.

The doctor quickly recognized these classic signs of diabetes. The boy was hospitalized and treated with insulin and intravenous fluids. Within twenty-four hours he was looking and feeling better. And his frequency of urination had decreased to almost normal.

This case illustrates the sudden onset and rapid progression of symptoms typical in a Type I, insulin-dependent, diabetic.

From the time he starts feeling bad, the child's health deteriorates dramatically within two to three weeks. In fact, rare is the patient who suffers from these effects for more than six weeks before diagnosis is made.

Loss of weight is one of the first signs, sapping the child's strength and energy. Prior to weight loss, he will start to spill sugar into his urine. He does not know what is happening to him, but he knows that he is going to the bathroom a lot more than usual. Consequently, he is thirsty all the time. He is also constantly hungry. And, in spite of eating to satisfy this tremendous appetite, he continues to lose weight.

The development of Type I diabetes progresses so fast that parents usually notice right away that something serious is happening to their child. Often, however, this type of diabetes will show itself after an infection or a bad cold, so the parents may attribute the symptoms to influenza and may be slow to bring the child in for diagnosis and treatment. As a result of this delay, the child may fall into a coma—becoming unconscious due to ketoacidosis—before his parents take him to the doctor. It is not at all uncommon for children to be brought into an emergency room in that state, even the children of diabetics, who may have difficulty accepting the possibility that their child has inherited a tendency to develop diabetes.

Searching for a Cause

In Type I diabetics, as mentioned in Chapter 2, most or all of the insulin-producing beta cells in the pancreas have been destroyed. What destroys these cells is still open to question. However, the destruction is thought to be the result of some kind of auto-immune response. Many studies have shown that antibodies to the beta cells can be detected in the blood months and years *before* the symptoms of Type I diabetes appear.

Curiously, there seems to be a seasonal trend for the onset of Type I diabetes. Doctors diagnose more cases of this disease in autumn and winter than at any other time of year. This trend has led researchers to suspect that the destruction of the beta cells might be caused by a variety of viral infections. Because the onset often happens in the cold and flu season, parents may mistake their child's severe symptoms as flu.

Those who support the virus theory believe that the infection is one to which most of the population is exposed sometime early in life. Most people, they hypothesize, recover from the infection without lasting ill effects. A few others, however, suffer the destruction of their beta cells and become Type I diabetics. The operating principle behind this theory is that the individual who develops Type I diabetes has had an abnormal immune response to a viral infection. His immune system produces cells and antibodies that not only destroy the virus but attack the beta cells as well. The immune response in another person with the same viral infection would destroy the virus alone (the normal reaction) leaving the beta cells unharmed.

Genetic Susceptibility

If a person has not developed Type I diabetes by the time he reaches maturity, proposes the theory, he has probably at some time come in contact with the virus and survived unharmed. Whether he has built up an immunity is still open to question. Recent studies indicate that the person who develops Type I diabetes has a genetic susceptibility to make immune cells and antibodies that will cross-react with the infecting virus and the beta cells while other people make immune cells and antibodies that *react only with* this virus. If the condition has not developed in a given individual by age twenty, chances are very good that it will not develop at all. (There are occasional instances in which people do fall prey to Type I diabetes late in life, but they are the exception to the rule.)

We do know that there are several "age peaks" at which Type I diabetes usually shows up. The first peak is shortly after birth.

The second peak falls around age two to three; the third at age seven to eight. The final and most common time of onset is just before puberty.

The "Honeymoon" Stage

An important footnote to our portrait of the Type I diabetic involves the rare—but well-described—case in which the patient, after being diagnosed, recovers enough to be declared nondiabetic. To put this kind of "miracle cure" in perspective, we must stress that in most Type I diabetics, all the beta cells *are not* destroyed at once. What happens, then, is that shortly after the newly diagnosed diabetic begins insulin treatment, he goes through a "honeymoon stage" in which the illness becomes much less severe. Usually these individuals will still require some insulin, but not nearly as much as they did when their diabetes was first diagnosed. Most often in these cases, their condition relapses soon thereafter, and they again require more insulin.

Some physicians suggest that this phenomenon is due to a temporary restoration of function in the few remaining beta cells. These cells, they point out, were overworked and exhausted by continually high blood glucose levels. But then, when the patient started insulin injections, his blood glucose levels were normalized and the surviving beta cells had a chance to recuperate and regain their capability to produce insulin, so the requirement for insulin injections decreased accordingly.

But at this point, if the destruction of these remaining beta cells continues, more insulin will be required. Whatever the reason, the important thing to remember is that an apparent reversal in such individuals is rarely, if ever, permanent.

The Type II Diabetic

Only 10–15 percent of all diabetics are Type I. As we have seen, the individual who develops this type of diabetes is most often a child and a victim of circumstances beyond his control or that of his parents. The disease strikes quickly, demanding immediate medical attention.

Type II (non-insulin-dependent) diabetes is quite another story. Its emergence, for one thing, is far more subtle than that of Type I, because there may be no dramatic changes at first. The typical victims of Type II are well past childhood, usually over the age of forty. Most of them, perhaps 80–90 percent, are overweight.

Type II diabetes develops gradually, and its victims may not even be certain there is anything wrong. They may have minimal symptoms for many years before the diagnosis is made.

Once the blood sugar level for these people is controlled—brought down to reasonably normal (70–120 mg/dl) or below 150 mg/dl—they recognize how much better they feel.

Occasionally, symptoms are obvious. A person may come to realize that he is urinating much more than he used to, that he has to get up at night to go to the bathroom and have a drink of water. He may feel so weak that he does not have the energy to do much of anything. Others have blurred or double vision (a symptom that occurs most often in older people).

Sometimes these people will get more infections than usual—particularly bladder or urinary tract infections—because the sugar in their urine makes them more susceptible to infection. For women, the excess sugar makes a favorable medium for the growth of fungus or yeast and bacteria, and so may result in vaginal infections as well. Vaginal and urinary tract infections, in fact, are frequently the symptoms through which a woman's doctor will discover that she has diabetes.

Poorly controlled diabetics, in general, are much more susceptible than others to developing infections from any kind of injury. However, if their blood sugar levels are controlled, such infections usually will heal normally. There is no evidence that healing will be impaired in a well-controlled diabetic who is free of vascular disease. We'll talk more about special health concerns for diabetics in Chapter 5.

A Matter of Degree

Another problem for doctors trying to diagnose Type II diabetes is that this disease can be present in different degrees. After undergoing various tests, you might ask your doctor, "Well, do I have it?" and expect a simple yes or no. As the discussion of blood sugar levels suggests, "normal" may vary from one person to the next. In addition, some individuals have elevated blood sugar only during times of stress, infection, or surgery. Why only at these times? Part of the answer may be that stress hormones produced in the adrenal glands alter overall body metabolism, including that of glucose. (We'll talk more about that in Chapter 16.)

So it is possible to discover that you have only a mild case, what some doctors used to call "borderline" diabetes. This diagnosis means that your blood sugar level is minimally but consistently above normal. Many of the people who hear this verdict are overweight. Compared to the established fasting norm of 115 mg/dl (milligrams of sugar in 1 deciliter of blood), an overweight person whose fasting level is between 125 and 140 mg/dl would be considered diabetic: but if he lost as little as five or ten pounds, his blood sugar level might well return to normal. Sometimes all that's required to achieve this normalization is a change in the timing and the size of his meals; he'll consume the same total number of calories, but instead of, say, a small breakfast and lunch followed by one big evening meal, he'll begin eating three small meals and three snacks a day. This change in habit spreads out the absorption of sugars from the intestines, thus keeping blood sugar closer to normal as well as helping him lose weight.

Doctors have weight-height charts that indicate the ideal weight for a given person of a certain height and sex. And anyone who purchases clothes off the rack knows that those model people must exist; clothing manufacturers seem to make most of the good-looking clothes for those rare perfect types.

The problem is that most of us are not perfect in every way. How do we deal with being overweight and being diagnosed as diabetic, whether borderline or clear-cut? We tend to think that physicians will have some magical cure or diet to make us thin and healthy again.

Well, that rarely happens. However, it does not always take magic or miracles to get the job done.

A Typical Type II Diabetic

A pastry truck driver came in for treatment. He weighed 220 pounds and was 5′6″ tall. For his height, he should have weighed approximately 152 pounds. In conversation, the patient revealed his daily routine:

He ate pastries in the morning before going to work. On the job, he had coffee and doughnuts. At lunch, he ate two hamburgers, french fries, and a sugared soft drink. When he went home in the evening, he took the leftover pastries with him for a snack. Perhaps 80 percent of his diet consisted of quick sugars (sugars that are rapidly absorbed raise blood sugar levels drastically and quickly). His blood glucose level was sometimes as high as 300 mg/dl.

If he were to require insulin injections, he feared his employer would not allow him to drive a truck. Because this job was important to him, he agreed to follow a prescribed weight-reduction program to the letter. He was started on an exercise program and a 1,500-calories-a-day diet, which he followed religiously. In ten days his blood sugar dropped to normal. While not everyone can expect to experience such a dramatic improvement in such a short time, it can happen.

As long as a person's blood sugar levels remain within the established normal range, he is obviously not considered diabetic. However, if he is overweight, common sense as well as medical knowledge dictates that he should try to lose weight. It isn't just a matter of blood sugar; a fat person (diabetic or nondiabetic) who slims down will feel better, improve his carbohydrate tolerance, reduce the work load on his heart, and may even lower blood pressure and blood fats.

Other Factors

The Type II diabetic frequently achieves his state as a consequence of being overweight often due to overeating, yet clearly, not all overweight people are diabetics. Nor are all Type II diabetics fat. So let's return to the pancreas and the genes to see what's going on.

If we examine the beta cells of a Type II diabetic, we will probably find not only that he has a lot of them but also that those cells may very well be filled with insulin.* For some reason, however, they are not able to release that insulin in response to the normal stimulus, which is an increase in the blood glucose level (and in certain amino acids) from the food eaten. The beta cells simply cannot manufacture and release enough insulin to keep sugar levels in the normal range, meaning that the pancreas cannot keep pace with the amount of food consumed. As we get older, there may be some slight impairment of insulin secretion or loss of insulin reserve. It is not clear how much these factors influence the onset of diabetes.

The importance of body weight is clearly demonstrated by people who can go back and forth between being diabetic or nondiabetic by losing or gaining as little as five to ten pounds. If

*It is worth mentioning that the total number or mass of insulin-producing beta cells in Type II diabetics is less than that found in nondiabetics. Whether these diabetics started life with fewer beta cells than normal or had the right number to begin with and then somehow lost them is not known.

they take the weight off, they are all right. If they put it back on, they are in trouble again. There is certainly no reason to think that the number of insulin-producing beta cells changes as their weight bounces back and forth, or that the size of the insulin reserve makes a crucial difference within such a small weight range. It appears, rather, that such people become more or less resistant to the effects of insulin according to the fluctuations in their weight. As their weight goes up, so does extra body fat which is known to increase insulin resistance, making ever more fervent demands on the pancreas. Current research is looking hard at this situation trying to determine what processes are involved.

The Diabetic Thin Person and the Nondiabetic Fat Person

In a recent study, four types of individuals were categorized according to the ability of their beta cells to release insulin in response to large amounts of sugar consumed. Those tested included nondiabetic and diabetic thin people and nondiabetic and diabetic fat people. Researchers monitored each subject to see how much insulin his pancreas would release into the blood after he drank a certain amount of sugar-containing beverage. They found that a nondiabetic thin person produced a lot more insulin in response to the increase in his blood sugar than the diabetic thin person, and that the same held true for the nondiabetic fat person in relation to the diabetic fat person.

But equally important in that study was the finding that the nondiabetic fat person produced far more insulin than the nondiabetic thin person. Subsequently, it was discovered that night and day the fat nondiabetic's insulin levels were higher than those of the thin nondiabetic. Researchers concluded that the fat person has to have a lot more insulin circulating to keep his blood glucose levels normal.

We really do not understand why obesity makes cells resistant to insulin. But we know that the body tries to compensate by making more insulin. That increased production of insulin, however, sets up what appears to be a vicious cycle.

Insulin Resistance

For some reason, higher blood insulin levels apparently cause a reduction in the number of insulin-receptor sites (areas on the cells which chemically attract or "bind" insulin) to which insulin would normally attach enabling those cells to metabolize nutrients. This is called "down regulation." Consequently, even though more insulin is released into the blood, less and less of it can bind to the cells that need it. That phenomenon is known as *insulin resistance* (Figure 1).

You can see the cycle here: As the number of receptors decreases, the cell becomes more and more resistant to insulin, and the pancreas produces an increasing amount of insulin (or

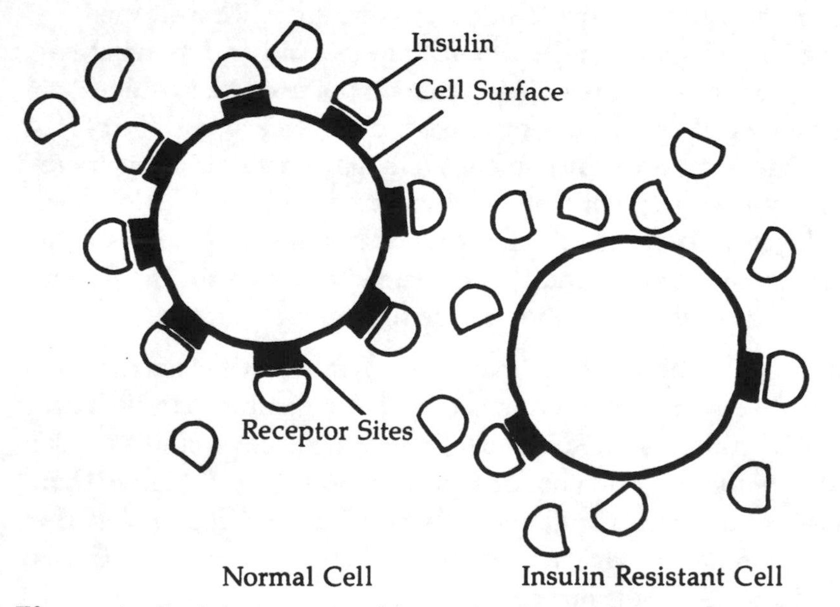

Figure 1 Resistance to insulin can be due to *decreased numbers* of insulin receptors.

tries to). The more insulin the pancreas produces, the more resistant the cells become, and so on. The cells seem to "know" that the body is too fat and are trying to reduce their uptake of nutrients even though the person keeps overeating.

When Insulin Does Not Bind

Another cause of Type II diabetes may be a condition in which the pancreas puts out enough insulin and the target cells have enough receptors, but the insulin does not bind properly to those receptors (Figure 2). Consequently, the insulin cannot act on the cells that need it to accept glucose. When, as a result, blood sugar levels rise above normal, other cells—those that do not need insulin to utilize glucose—now have high sugar levels. These cells become damaged, leading to further health complications. The main victims here are the cells that line the blood vessel walls, kidneys and the nervous system.

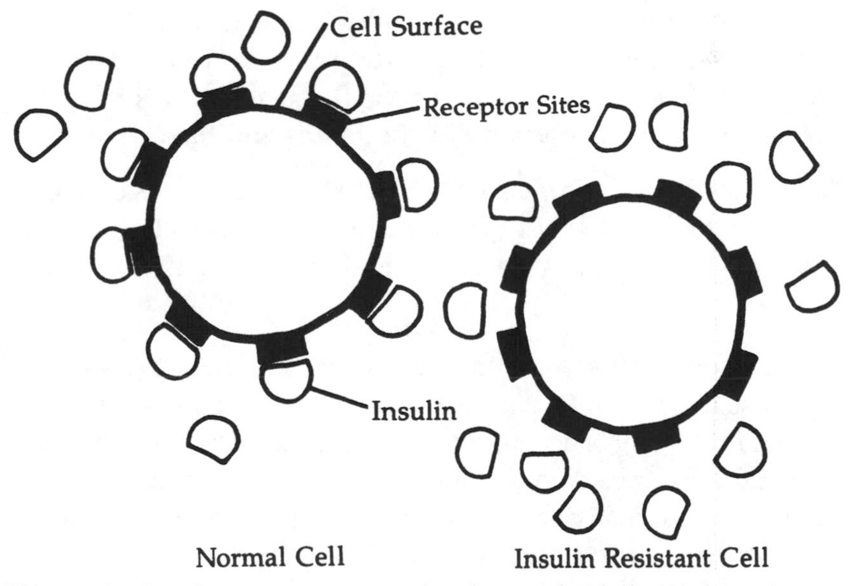

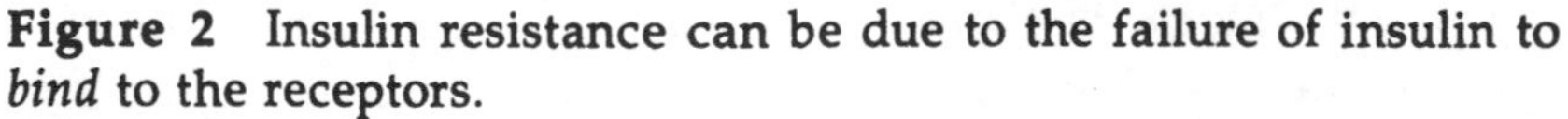

Figure 2 Insulin resistance can be due to the failure of insulin to *bind* to the receptors.

Secondary Diabetes

Almost any disease or drug that decreases glucose uptake by tissues or increases glucose output by the liver or induces insulin resistance will end up causing high blood sugar. By definition that is considered to be diabetes. But if the underlying disease or treatment causing high blood glucose is recognized, the diabetes can be accounted for by that factor rather than by the hereditary factors typically responsible for Type I and Type II diabetes.

Diabetes caused by such an "outside" factor is known as secondary diabetes. This type is usually mild and not insulin-dependent (except when the aggravating condition involves destruction of the pancreas).

One of the diseases that typically leads to secondary diabetes is acromegaly, a disorder in which the pituitary produces an overabundance of growth hormone. This condition is most often caused by a tumor in the pituitary gland, which produces the growth hormone. The excess growth hormone causes thickening of the bones and coarsening of the features, a change in head shape, and enlargement of the hands and feet.

The excess growth hormone also stimulates insulin production while decreasing the responsiveness of the cells that use insulin. As a result, blood levels of both glucose and insulin are elevated.

Another condition associated with secondary diabetes is Cushing's disease, which is caused by excess production of adrenal corticoid or glucocorticoid hormones. Like acromegaly, this disorder may be traced to a tumor situated, in this case, in the pituitary or adrenal glands. Glucocorticoids are steroids that affect cellular metabolism, basically promoting the breakdown of muscle and interfering with the ability of cells to use glucose. Therefore, a surplus of glucocorticoids (which may occur during infections, stressful situations or during steroid treatment) will cause blood glucose to rise because the target cells cannot use it. In addition, amino acids formed by the breakdown of muscle cells are transported to the liver, where they are converted to glucose. So, again, the sum total is a decrease in glucose utilization and an increase in its production.

Diabetes may also result from chronic pancreatitis. Pancreatitis means inflammation of the pancreas, and is sometimes caused by tumors in that region of the body. Often, so much of the pancreas is destroyed that there are not enough beta cells left to meet the demand for insulin. In addition, the pancreas may not make enough digestive enzymes to digest the food consumed.

Cystic fibrosis also leads to extensive destruction of the pancreas and, therefore, may destroy beta cells. Thus, diabetes is common in people with cystic fibrosis.

An unusual disease called *hemochromatosis* may also cause secondary diabetes. This disease is most common in older men whose intestinal tract absorbs too much iron. Iron deposits accumulate in the beta cells as well as elsewhere in the body and, for reasons not understood, impair function, so diabetes develops.

The Potential Diabetic

A person who was once a diabetic is always a potential diabetic. And if a nondiabetic person with carbohydrate intolerance overeats on quick sugars, his blood glucose levels may shoot up dangerously high at isolated times, even though they are generally within the normal range. Eventually, he may suffer the same long-term complications that a chronic diabetic will.

It all depends on the ability of one's pancreas to make and release insulin. If the pancreas has a consistently ample reserve of insulin, then it can put out enough to metabolize all the sugar from a sweet soft drink, for instance, without letting blood glucose levels rise. But what about the fellow who has normal blood sugar levels under a strict diet but whose beta cells store only a marginal quantity of insulin? If he consumes that same sweet soft drink, his pancreas may not be able to handle it, and the effects of elevated blood glucose levels on his body may be harmful and permanent. Eventually, diabetes will develop and oral medication or insulin will be required to control blood sugar.

Every person's body reacts differently; that's why diabetes is so difficult to treat. The more we learn, the more we realize how important early diagnosis, proper management, education, and patience are to helping the diabetic lead a long, full life.

CHAPTER 4

Living an Active, Healthier Life

In the last section of this book, we will lay out what we consider to be the best, most up-to-date methods of treatment for diabetes—methods we have put into practice with positive results. Before we continue our discussion of diabetes itself and its varying effects on our lives—some of which may strike you as grim indeed—it seems appropriate to address, just briefly, *how much can be done* to stave off those grim effects.

It is so easy, as we've pointed out, to deny a chronic illness—or to tell oneself that the worst is inevitable, that treatment is too complicated and useless anyway, and to recklessly throw all caution to the wind. But learning to live with diabetes is not as hard as you may imagine. In some ways, it's a lot easier than having to share your home with an ill-tempered relative—an analogous situation of sorts, the difference being that you *can* get the upper hand on diabetes.

Under the proper treatment program, a diabetic can do almost everything a nondiabetic can do, except when it comes to diet. Of course, as soon as something like a candy bar or a sugared soft drink is declared "forbidden fruit," that's exactly what we crave. But consider this: If you were handed a bottle marked "Delicious Poison," you would no more consider sampling the contents than you would opt to go blind. However, if a diabetic does not control the excess sugar in his blood, that may be the literal choice he (or she) is facing: to resist temptation or to go blind or develop other serious complications. The diabetic's number one goal is to normalize his blood glucose level all twenty-four hours of the day. This is achieved not just through insulin supplements—even with added insulin, a diabetic can still have high blood sugar—but through improved diet and exercise habits as well.

Who Must Take Insulin?

As you have already learned, the Type I diabetic's pancreas no longer produces insulin, or produces so little that he or she is dependent upon insulin shots for survival. "Well," you say, "I can see why that Type I diabetic has to take insulin, but I'm a Type II. My beta cells have not been destroyed. Why should I need to take insulin?"

The reality is that many Type II diabetics do have to take insulin. Although only 10 percent or so of the diabetic population is Type I, approximately 50 percent of *all* diabetics are treated with insulin. This means close to half of all Type II's require treatment that includes regular insulin injections. The need for extra insulin is dictated purely by an individual's degree of insulin insufficiency, not by the particular "Type" of diabetes.

The Type I diabetic takes insulin because his body's production of the hormone is insignificant or nonexistent and he cannot live without it. With the Type II individual, the reasons for taking insulin are more complicated; the need for insulin depends on several factors, namely:

- Body weight and amount of body fat;
- The rate at which the pancreas can produce and release insulin;
- The size of the insulin reserve;
- The number of insulin receptors on the target cells; and
- The presence of kidney or liver disease.

If you are a Type II diabetic, your doctor will conduct tests to determine as accurately as possible the interrelationships of these factors in your particular case. And he just might decide that, at least to begin with, insulin is an essential part of the proper regimen for you.

You may find this prospect depressing or frightening. But you will be surprised to find out how quickly this part of treatment becomes routine. Even athletes can make insulin injections (by syringe or insulin pump) a part of their everyday regimen without compromising their active lifestyle.

Oral Agents

For some Type II diabetics, oral agents—medications taken by mouth—are an alternative to insulin treatment. These drugs do a number of things to help the pancreas perform its job provided there are enough beta cells still there. The first oral agents were discovered by French medical investigators doing research on antibiotics. They found that some of their laboratory animals were becoming hypoglycemic (low blood sugar) after taking certain medications on a regular basis. Eventually, it occurred to the researchers that these medications were promoting the release of insulin from the pancreas—a side effect that could be an obvious benefit to the Type II diabetic. Not every patient, however, is a candidate for oral agents, and their use generally calls for extra monitoring on the part of the physician and following a proper diet by the patient. The oral medications available today are safe and effective when they are used properly.

We'll discuss oral agents and other new methods of insulin treatment more thoroughly in Chapters 14 and 17.

Exercise and Diet

The vast majority of Type II diabetics are over age forty and are overweight. While nothing can be done about being over forty, being overweight is quite another matter.

Which brings us to the topic of exercise and diet. As you probably know, exercise stimulates blood circulation and peps up metabolism. These effects are beneficial to just about everybody; they may be especially so for the diabetic, since they facilitate the uptake of vital nutrients (including glucose and amino acids) by the tissues.

Exercise has an effect that, apparently, opens the pores on the membranes of muscle cells and lets in nutrients in a way that actually *minimizes* the need for insulin. This effect has yet to be fully explained, but it is well documented. It enables the muscles to take up nutrients more efficiently and to increase their mass if enough insulin is available.

However, it is important to note that exercise is *not* recommended for diabetics who are not under proper treatment to control blood sugar and insulin levels, because exercise without adequate insulin acts as a stress on the body and leads to increased levels of glucose in the blood, free fatty acids and ketones—which, as we've seen, can cause ketoacidosis.

The Right Kind of Exercise

Different individuals benefit from different forms of exercise. Choosing the right kind involves considering, mainly, one's age and general state of health. For diabetics with coronary artery disease, for instance, or those well up in years, the most appropriate exercise is probably brisk walking, or riding a stationary bicycle, or some similar exercise that doesn't put unnecessary strain on the heart and joints.

For others—those who are younger, active, generally vigorous, and show no signs of cardiovascular disease—swimming is one of the best all-around exercises.

Jogging is good exercise for someone young and energetic, but it puts an unnecessary hardship on the body. When a person jogs, he subjects his ankles, knees, and hips to repeated impact, thus risking physical stress and even injury.

Various competitive sports may be beneficial, too. The main thing to remember is that you must find the exercise that's a wise choice for *you;* seeking your doctor's advice in this health matter, as in all others, is a good idea. We highly recommend self blood glucose monitoring before and after exercise.

Diet: The Dreaded Word

Diet does not have to create the great dread it often does for the overweight person. A considerate doctor or diabetes nurse educator will find out what foods a patient likes, then work out a diet that incorporates the foods from that list that are lowest in calories. In this way a diabetic trying to lose weight may even be able to "splurge" on a particular favorite food while minimizing calorie intake.*

The physician who works with diabetics should never simply hand out a predetermined diet and say, "This is what you have to eat." He or his nurse educator or dietitian should develop a personalized diet for every patient, based on individual taste or ethnic preferences and budget limitations.

---

*See list of cookbooks in the Appendix.

A diabetic also needs to adapt his all-around lifestyle to his diet. He should strive to eat his meals at approximately the same time seven days a week (basically a good habit for anyone).

A Word about Fasting

Any proper diet involves regular meals. Fasting, which some people think will achieve the same results in a shorter period of time, is detrimental to the body. This is especially true for diabetics, whose metabolism is handicapped to begin with. Normally, if you fast for a period of twenty-four hours, all the glycogen that you have stored away in the liver will be used up. When that happens and the brain needs sugar, the amino acids which are normally and continually released from muscle cells into the blood, as described in Chapter 2, are transformed by the liver into glucose to supply the brain with its fuel. (The body has no reserve storage depot for amino acids as it does for sugar.)

Someone on a fast will thus lose muscle mass and strength as well as fat, especially if not exercising. In order to regain that strength, it is necessary to rebuild muscle. A person should always diet in such a way that overall food intake is reduced enough that body fat stores are burned, while enough carbohydrates and proteins are eaten to maintain muscle mass.

The principles are basic:

1. If you need insulin to survive, there is no substitute. You must take it, whether by injection, insulin pump, or some other means.
2. Exercise is important for the diabetic—as it is for everyone. Choose a form that is comfortable and healthy for *you*.

3. A controlled diet is essential, but the diabetic does not by any means have to give up all the foods he likes. You can enjoy eating and still maintain a healthy diet.

Pretty simple. What it all means is that if you have diabetes, you *can* live with it and still enjoy life. If you think this is too much trouble, read on. If you do not control this disease, the consequences to your body and your future can be disastrous.

CHAPTER 5

The Truth about the Consequences

"Too much of a good thing is wonderful," Mae West once said. That philosophy, however, does not apply to *all* good things.

There is no question that our body needs glucose. But give it too much and our system gets fouled up.* The same is true for cholesterol, which is an essential component in the membranes of every cell in our body. There is no way we can survive without it. However, when the concentrations in the blood are too high, cholesterol poses a serious hazard to our well-being.

To be blunt, the potential health problems facing a diabetic who does not follow a proper course of treatment are catastrophic. They include:

*Some controversy still exists over the question of how much direct damage is done to the body by high blood sugar. We'll discuss that controversy when we talk about the state of diabetes research in Part II. But we feel confident that our viewpoint—as laid out in this book—is firmly supported by the most recent medical discoveries.

Cardiovascular disease
Stroke
Peripheral arterial disease
Gangrene
Kidney disease
Blindness
Hypertension
Nerve damage
Impotence
Increased incidence of infection
Loss of muscle mass and strength
Gastrointestinal dysfunction
Stiffness of joints and skin
Decreased color discrimination

One of the difficulties in discussing serious diseases is that most of us are unable or unwilling to contemplate them as being real until they hit us personally. Still, they *are* real, and one reason we flounder in trying to understand them is that we tend to think of them only in their tragic finality, envisioning ourselves as hopelessly disabled and withering away. This is pure melodrama. If this is your state of mind, force yourself to imagine instead the continuation—even the improvement—of your life, once you've become accustomed to a treatment that will *save* your life.

What we are going to do in this chapter is to explain what can happen in the body of the uncontrolled or poorly controlled diabetic that sets the stage and leads to the previously listed catastrophes.

Strengths and Weaknesses of Our Cardiovascular System

Every day of our lives, every hour twenty-four hours a day, the heart pumps about forty gallons of blood through our blood vessels. The heart is a very efficient pump, considering that it works continually for about seventy years. But no matter how good it is, the heart suffers normal wear and tear.

All of the blood vessels in our body are elastic. But that elasticity is limited, and if the pressure at any point is too great, a vessel can burst. Over the years, just as part of the normal aging process, the elasticity is reduced, just as the elastic in a bathing suit wears out with time.

We tend to think of everything in our bodies as being fixed in place. In a sense that is true. Our parts do not go wandering all over. However, the large vessels coming out of the heart do move as the blood is pumped through them. These vessels are subject to bending and stretching at the junctions where smaller vessels branch off. Consequently, in the normal course of events, these large arteries of the vascular system are constantly being "injured" by this stress. The body makes scar tissue to repair the injury.

Scar Tissue Versus Cell Regeneration

Some tissues and cells can regenerate in response to injury—lost cells are actually replaced by new ones. As an example, when you cut yourself, scar tissue forms. However, over the surface of the scar tissue the epidermis (skin) will regenerate and cover the repair. The cells lining the intestinal tract are continually being replaced because of normal wear. The liver tissue also can regenerate.

Other cells in the body do not have this ability. Neither the heart nor the brain, for instance, can replace lost or damaged cells. The same holds true once a certain amount of damage has been done to some of the blood vessels. They cannot be replaced, and all that is left to maintain the continuity of the vessel wall is scar tissue.

Scar tissue needs to last a long time and it does. However, it is not elastic. Where there is scar tissue, the vessels are less elastic and less movable. As a result, the stress is transmitted to the adjacent parts of the vessel that are still elastic. This causes more injury, and more scar tissue is formed. Badly scarred vessels do not function normally. They are like stiff pipes and cannot dilate to carry more blood or constrict to decrease blood flow.

This whole scarring process accelerates when we have high blood pressure, or when the levels of cholesterol or sugar in the blood become too high. Any combination of the three further speeds up the cycle of injury, scarring, and strain on adjacent tissue. Cigarette smoking is another major contributor to this damage.

How Vessels Become Leaky

The forty gallons of blood being pumped through the heart every hour sends a lot of traffic through the aorta, the artery which carries all of the blood leaving the heart. Potentially, it may have to cope with more problems than it is equipped to handle.

The aorta branches off into many smaller vessels, which carry blood to all the different organs of the body. The largest branches of the aorta, some of which are important enough to have individual names, are the arteries. The smallest vessels are the capillaries, which split off from the small arteries. The blood is carried from the capillaries back to the heart by the veins.

Lining the inside of the aorta and all the other vessels are endothelial cells that abut one another like bricks in a wall. When high blood sugar, high cholesterol, and high blood pressure or cigarette smoking—separately or in combination—damage these cells, the cells separate and this inner lining of the vessel walls becomes leaky. Then cholesterol, normally present in the blood, seeps into the walls, where it accumulates and causes additional damage to muscle cells in the vessel wall interior. When that happens, the muscle cells respond by making scar tissue. Unfortunately, the excess scar tissue further interferes with the ability of the muscle cells to contract and regulate blood flow and can eventually build up enough to block off the vessel.

High Blood Sugar and Sorbitol

Recent experiments have demonstrated that high blood sugar, independent of high blood pressure, excess cholesterol, or cigarette smoking, makes the vessels leaky. Remember that even if a person has normal cholesterol levels, that substance is nevertheless present, ready to enter a leaky vessel wall and wreak its damage. (Remember, also, that in uncontrolled diabetics, blood levels of fatty acids as well as glucose are increased. And, as described in Chapter 1, those fatty acids are converted by the liver to low-density lipoproteins—carriers of cholesterol.)

How high blood sugar causes the vessels to become leaky has not yet been precisely determined. Increasing evidence suggests that since the cells lining the vessels' interior do not require insulin for glucose uptake, too much glucose is getting inside those cells, and some of that excess is transformed into an unusual type of sugar alcohol called sorbitol, which accumulates inside the cells and damages them. Another theory is that metabolic imbalances associated with the formation of sorbitol, rather than sorbitol itself, may cause the injury. One of these metabolic imbalances associated with the formation of sorbitol is a loss of another type of sugar alcohol called myo-inositol which is vital to normal cell metabolism. Loss of myo-inositol has been implicated in nerve damage and cataract formation, as well as in vascular disease.

There is a lot of controversy over whether the sorbitol itself injures the cell or the injury is caused by the consequences of metabolic imbalances associated with sorbitol formation. In any case, recent studies of diabetic animals have shown:

1. Increased vascular leakage in the eyes, nerves and aorta is linked to increased formation of sorbitol from glucose.
2. Drugs which interfere with the accumulation of sorbitol do prevent cataracts as well as nerve damage and vascular injury.

Another possibility is that glucose is sticking to cell surfaces (glycosylation), interfering with the function of those cells and their ability to hang onto one another.

In any case, by whatever mechanisms, excess glucose injures blood vessel walls and nerves. There does not appear to be any safe "above normal" value at which one can be confident that such damage will not occur.

Various studies suggest that a person's likelihood of suffering vascular disease increases in proportion to blood glucose levels above normal. The practical conclusion we may draw from these findings is that *any reduction of blood glucose levels toward normal will reduce the long-term risk of vascular disease.*

Think about the average Type II diabetic. He is over forty and overweight. We know that he has high blood sugar. He probably has high cholesterol and he may even be at the upper ranges of normal blood pressure for his age. Even the upper ranges of "so-called" *normal* blood pressure may add to the damage, as will cigarette smoking. Because of these conditions, cholesterol is leaking into the vessel walls and producing injury and scar tissue at a much higher rate than normal.

How Bad Can It Get?

It is important to bear in mind that once extensive scar tissue has formed in arteries, it probably *cannot be reversed.* It is not like smoking and lung damage, where—up to a certain point—

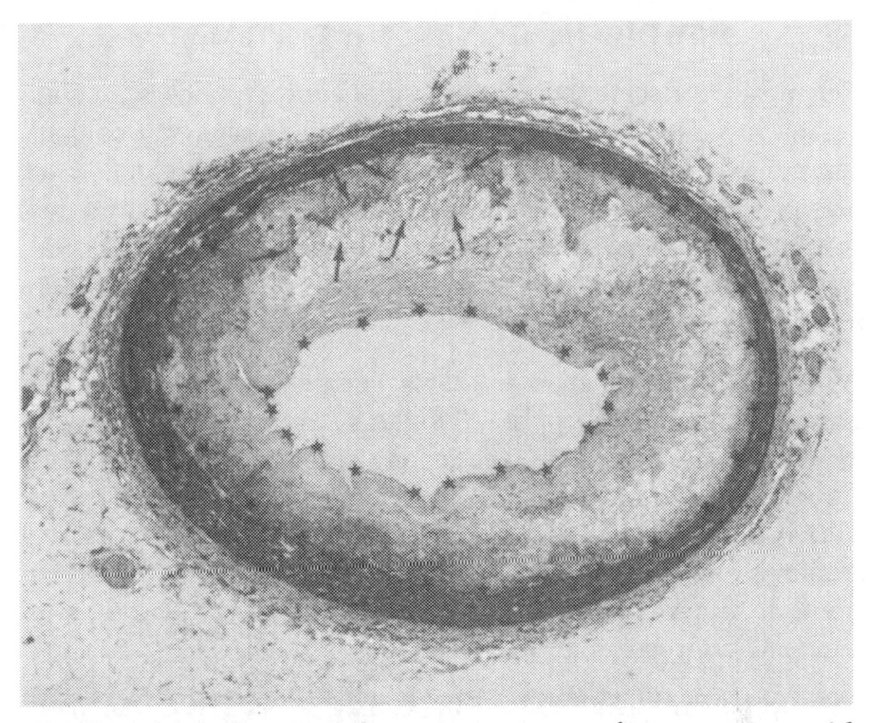

Figure 1 Cross-section of a coronary artery from a person with poorly controlled diabetes for 15 years. The photo shows marked accumulation of scar tissue (area between asterisks) and cholesterol deposits (arrows) which have narrowed the inside opening of the vessel by 75 percent.

a person who quits smoking can actually *renew* the quality of lung tissue.

For the diabetic, to delay initiation of the proper treatment regimen may contribute to the permanent physical destruction of the circulatory system. What is the worst that can happen? Well, when a damaged vessel of the heart collects cholesterol and scar tissue, it begins to close up (Figure 1). Once it gets too clogged or closes off completely, the person has a heart attack, which may be fatal. If the blocked-off vessel is in the brain, a stroke results—also sometimes fatal or resulting in paralysis. If it's in the leg, the blockage may lead to gangrene and require amputation.

Symptoms of Vascular Damage

The most worrisome aspect of vascular complications is that our vessels can sustain a lot of damage before causing any obvious symptoms. Without any warning, a person who thinks that he or she is healthy may have a heart attack or heart arrhythmia resulting in sudden death. By the time symptoms appear, vessels are already almost closed off and the damage may be irreversible.

When symptoms do show up early, they are usually the result of inadequate blood supply. When this happens in the heart, it may cause angina; in the legs it may cause pain after walking only short distances (technically known as claudication). When it happens in the brain, the person may become senile, have a stroke or have transient impairment of brain function (transient ischemic attacks or TIA's), weak spells, dizziness or experience problems with vision or balance.

These problems are all caused by damage to arteries. Damaged capillaries generally give rise to different symptoms. It appears, for instance, that scar-tissue buildup around these small vessels occurs earliest in the kidneys. It also occurs in the eyes, nerves, and legs.

When capillaries in a kidney are scarred, the units that filter waste products from the blood cease to function. Consequently, the kidney cannot get rid of body wastes and the person suffers renal failure, ultimately requiring a kidney transplant or dialysis program in order to live.

When circulation in any part of the body is impaired, the healing response will be slowed down and the chances of infection will be increased. (This is true for diabetics and nondiabetics alike.) The key to healing of any kind is increased blood flow. With vascular complications, the body may not be able to respond properly with an increase in blood flow and healing will be impaired.

Bad Nerves

When people talk about "bad nerves," they are usually referring to psychological behavior, i.e., nervousness. Bad nerves in a diabetic are more like electrical short circuits—a truly physiological problem.

The information transmitted by nerves—the ability to sense touch, pain, temperature, and so forth—is carried electrically. The nerve is like an electrical cord, and, like an electrical cord, it has to be insulated. Otherwise, the impulse shorts out and never gets to the brain, or is altered and creates strange sensations.

The nerve fibers that carry the electrical impulses (sensations of touch, pain, etc.) correspond to the wire in an electrical cord; the insulation around the nerve fibers is comprised of wrappings of Schwann cells. Both the nerve fibers and the Schwann cells are freely permeable to glucose—that is, glucose gets in easily without the aid of insulin. When glucose levels get too high, and too much is metabolized into sorbitol, both the nerve fibers and the Schwann cells are overloaded with this chemical and begin to degenerate. When this happens the nerve fibers can no longer conduct electrical impulses and the Schwann cells lose their ability to insulate. The result is like having broken wires and short circuits. This condition is called neuropathy.

Someone afflicted by neuropathy may experience bizarre sensations: for instance, tingling or numbness in the feet not unlike the feeling from being accidentally shocked. When the neuropathy has progressed further, the patient may not be able to tell when he steps on a rock or burns his foot. Or he may suffer from constant painful sensations. Many people with this condition are in constant misery and cannot sleep. This is sometimes the case with very poorly controlled diabetics.

Extreme Complications

A poorly controlled diabetic who drinks alcohol may face even worse complications where the nerves are concerned. Alcohol affects metabolism and is also soluble in lipids (fats).

The Schwann cells that insulate the nerves are composed largely of lipids. So alcohol may accumulate in the Schwann cells and intensify the damage done to these cells by high blood sugar. Diabetics who drink heavily appear to be especially prone to neuropathy (nerve damage).

And when both vascular and neurological disease affect the lower extremities, a person may have trouble healing injuries caused by trauma or infection. As an example, if a diabetic does not feel foot pain, he or she may walk with a pebble in a shoe for some time and develop a serious blister or ulcer (which can easily become infected) before he becomes aware of the problem. Because of the poor blood supply to the injured area, the diabetic may have trouble overcoming the infection, and it may take longer than usual for the wound to heal. The loss of sensation combined with poor blood supply sets the stage for gangrene and amputation.

Some guidelines to proper foot care for diabetics are:

- Wear comfortable, well-fitting shoes.
- Wash feet daily; dry thoroughly.
- Powder feet and shoes.
- Keep feet warm and dry.
- Wear loose-fitting socks to bed if feet are cold; never use hot packs or hot water bottles.
- Inspect feet regularly for cuts or blisters.
- Cut toenails straight across.
- Use a mild lubricant for cracking and drying.
- Inspect the inside of shoes for tears, objects or rough spots.

Diabetics should avoid:

- Walking barefoot, even indoors!
- Cutting corns or calluses yourself.
- Open-toed shoes, or shoes with straps between the toes.

The Risk of Blindness

The eye is really an extension of the brain. As such, it is part of the nervous system and behaves like nerve tissue. The early changes brought about by diabetic vascular disease take place in the smallest vessels, though it is not yet exactly clear what happens. We do know, however, that blood flow is increased and that little aneurysms in the capillaries are a characteristic early form of damage. These aneurysms are balloonlike swellings of the capillaries. Sometimes they disappear, but other times they rupture and bleed, causing partial or complete loss of vision.

In the diabetic, something, as yet unknown, triggers the formation of new vessels in the eye. These small vessels are very fragile and tend to bleed. When they bleed, scar tissue begins to form. One peculiar feature of scar tissue anywhere, be it on the skin or in the eye, is that as it matures, it shrinks.

In most places—if the scarred area is not too large—when it shrinks, it does not cause any problems. However, if a person gets burned over a large part of an arm, the scar tissue may shrink enough to cause deformities.

When scar tissue in the eye starts contracting, it pulls the retina off the back of the eye. The retina is where all the nerve endings are that enable a person to see. They are the sensors. Once the retina is pulled off, serious loss of vision will result if the condition is not treated immediately. Even before this happens, a person often will begin to have trouble seeing, since the hemorrhaging and the scarring will create opaque areas that interfere with vision.

That is why it is so important for a diabetic to have regular eye examinations; the doctor will want to pick up any evidence of these changes as early as possible. Fortunately, there are several procedures that can help seal off bleeding vessels and prevent scar formation and retinal detachment.

Muscle Starvation

Perhaps the most visible consequence of unchecked diabetes is muscle atrophy. Without adequate insulin, as we've said, the muscles cannot take up the necessary nutrients to maintain themselves. Thus they are effectively starved. If you examine the leg or hand muscles of a poorly controlled diabetic, you will see that often they are very thin. The diabetic's muscles are, in a very real sense, wasting away. Muscles may also atrophy (from disuse) if the nerves that normally stimulate them to contract are damaged (as described earlier in this chapter under, "Bad Nerves").

CHAPTER 6

Victims of Heredity and Environment

Many of our most profound scientific discoveries stem from the comparison of humans and mice. Most people are not aware of the remarkable similarity between humans and mice when it comes to genetics and metabolism. This is one reason mice are so valuable to medical research.

Like a fat person, for instance, a fat mouse is also a candidate for diabetes. Indeed, some of our ideas regarding the role of heredity in obesity and in diabetes were first suggested by laboratory studies on mice.

As you know, we inherit a mixture of genes from our mothers and fathers. That mixture provides the strengths and weaknesses of our physical makeup. The strengths we take for granted; it is the weaknesses that give us problems. Susceptibility to develop diabetes is one of those weaknesses. What about the susceptibility to develop the complications? Does that also depend on genes?

What the Figures Say

Usually, we will not quote statistics in this book. However, we are going to make an exception here, because of the continuing controversy regarding the role of hereditary factors in determining the onset of diabetic complications. Some medical researchers are convinced that complications of diabetes are genetically ordained and will occur regardless of whether high blood sugar is controlled, so why bother or worry about diet and trying to normalize blood sugar?

In 1985 the Carter Center of Emory University study of "The Problem of Diabetes Mellitus in the United States" published the following figures comparing the diabetic with the general population. Their findings (data is derived from studies and surveys performed by the National Center for Health Statistics) revealed that compared to the average nondiabetic, a diabetic is:

- 6.8 times more likely to become blind,
- 11.3 times more likely to develop kidney disease,
- 29.9 times more likely to get gangrene,
- 4.6 times more likely to develop heart disease, and
- 5.4 times more likely to have a stroke.

When the study was released, diabetes was ranked as the third leading cause of death in this country. But some experts claim it is even higher now, because diabetes contributes to heart disease, which is the number-one killer. People who die of heart disease and who also have carbohydrate intolerance or impaired glucose tolerance are not classified for statistical purposes as diabetic, even though those conditions obviously could have contributed to the heart disease.

It is now estimated that diabetes is a significant factor in at least 134,000 deaths a year in the United States, and that 600,000 new cases of diabetes are diagnosed every year.* The number of people with diabetes increases by more than 6 percent per year. At that rate, the number of diabetics diagnosed will double every fifteen years.

Obesity and Predisposition

If that seems like an outrageous prediction, consider the Pima Indians of the Southwest. In this group, more than half of the adult population is diabetic. A disproportionately high segment of the population is also obese; and, as we've shown, this characteristic in itself makes one a prime candidate for Type II diabetes. A very high frequency of obesity along with diabetes has been observed in several other tribes of Indians as well.

This high frequency of obesity is generally blamed on the relatively sedentary lifestyle of these tribes. And if we compare these populations to the American people as a whole—with their increasingly relaxed way of life—the projections of a very high frequency of diabetes in American people as a whole are not as farfetched as they may at first sound.

Let's return to the mouse. Like humans, the mouse has a genetic code that determines its physical makeup. We are a long way from breaking that code. However, there is strong evidence that genetic makeup predisposes certain mice to being fat. What is not yet clear is whether that fat is the result of their eating in response to a constant hunger or simply of their being less physically active than other strains of mice. At any rate, these fat mice are especially prone to diabetes.

Susceptibility to Type II

Two factors appear to be influential in developing Type II diabetes. One is genetic susceptibility; the second is overeating.

*At present the annual health-care costs for diabetes exceed 14 billion dollars. See *Diabetes in America: Diabetes Data,* compiled 1984.

The exact nature of the susceptibility component for Type II diabetes is not well understood. It may be a gene that limits pancreatic insulin reserve, or one that might affect metabolism in such a way that if a person consumes excess calories and becomes obese, he or she will then develop diabetes.

So it is with the Pima Indians. The combination of genes and obesity leads to diabetes. Among this group there is a definite familial tendency to develop Type II diabetes; often many members of the same family are overweight and diabetic.

However, if all we had to go on was this familial tendency to develop Type II diabetes, it would really be difficult to know for certain whether the tendency was due to genetic factors or if it occurred in part because the family shared the same eating habits or had all been exposed to the same infection. What enables us to rule out the idea of infection is that when these people lose weight, their diabetes often disappears. This means that the diabetes had to do with how much food was being eaten or the type of food eaten. And since there are families of people and of mice who consume the same number of calories and are obese but not diabetic, that tells us that the susceptibility of obese people to develop Type II diabetes is determined by hereditary factors *coupled* with overeating. It comes down to insulin reserve in the pancreas. The quantity of that reserve is probably in large part genetically determined.

Susceptibility to Type I

The role of genetic factors as determinants of susceptibility to developing Type I diabetes is much clearer. Some strains of mice are susceptible to developing diabetes through viruses. If these mice are infected with certain viruses, a high proportion of them suffer damage to their beta cells and will become diabetic. When other strains of mice are infected with the same viruses, they do not become diabetic.

So it is clear from such studies that the susceptibility to become a diabetic after infection with a virus is genetically determined. The conclusion we have been able to draw from such studies is that two factors are required for development of diabetes associated with viral infections. The first is hereditary susceptibility, and the second, of course, is being infected with the virus. This may be one explanation for development of Type I diabetes in humans.

Evidence from Human Genetics

Studies of identical twins, who have exactly the same genes, uphold the theory that the genes involved in Type I and Type II diabetes are different. It is well-known that among identical twins, if one twin develops Type II diabetes, the other twin will almost certainly follow suit within a few years.

On the other hand, if one twin develops Type I diabetes, the other has only about a 50 percent chance of developing it within the next few years, and if he or she still does not have it after five to 10 years have passed, chances are that individual is at minimal risk to develop Type I diabetes.

In view of the fact that identical twins have identical genes, the simplest explanation for the finding that one can be diabetic while the other is not is that the twin with diabetes must have been exposed to some environmental factor—such as a virus or overeating—to which the nondiabetic twin was *not* exposed.

Type I and the Immune Response

The hereditary nature of Type I diabetes was discovered as an outgrowth of another study. Scientists were typing human leukocyte antigens (molecules that induce immune responses) for research in transplant surgery, determining the type of antigens carried by individuals in order to correctly match the antigens of donor organs to those of the recipients. If a match is not correct, the recipient's body will reject the organ.

The researchers discovered that several diseases were associated with particular kinds of antigens. Then they discovered that certain antigens were unusually common in the Type I (but not in the Type II) diabetic. Since antigens are genetically determined, it was clear that genetic factors do play a role in determining who will develop Type I diabetes, and that these factors differ from those that predispose someone to Type II.

Some researchers suspect that susceptibility to Type I diabetes, however, is related not to the leukocyte antigens but, rather, to the genes that regulate immune responses, which happen to be situated so near the genes for leukocyte antigens that they are often inherited together as a package (i.e., on the same chromosome). Thus one can be fairly certain that someone who shows an abundance of those antigens will also have an abnormal immune response. Consequently, when that individual is infected with a virus, the immune system apparently does not respond appropriately, and that leads to the destruction of the beta cells, which leads to diabetes.

On the basis of this information, if families were tested and someone was found to have these particular leukocyte antigens, it could be predicted that that individual would be at high risk for Type I diabetes—as would be his or her descendants if they inherited the same antigens, whether or not that particular person actually developed the illness.

New studies are underway to search for similar "lab markers" that would indicate Type II predisposition as well. Already these studies suggest that genes may actually determine the capacity of the beta cells to produce insulin.

Responding to the Environment

All these various studies show, if you read between the lines, that whether one develops diabetes is not simply a matter of genes. Look, for instance, at the pairs of identical twins in which only *one* develops this chronic disease. What about outside factors, our physical and behavioral environment?

In a syposium on diabetes in Israel in the winter of 1982, one of the topics discussed was what medicine has learned from animal models of diabetes. Of particular interest is a species of desert rat that survives quite well in its harsh environment where food is scarce. However, when the animal is placed in a situation where food is plentiful, it will develop a form of diabetes that corresponds to Type II diabetes in humans.

It is clear that not all animals respond this way. However, there is a parallel in human society. In Europe during both world wars, when food was scarce, large numbers of people lost a lot of weight, and the frequency of diabetes dropped. After each war, when food once more became plentiful, a sizable portion of the population again became fat—and diabetic. From these historical instances alone, we can see the importance of an environmental factor (i.e., the amount of food consumed), independent of genetic factors, in precipitating diabetes. In fact, overeating may well be the predominant environmental factor contributing to diabetes. Remember that over the ages humans have developed an amazingly efficient system of processing and conserving energy. Constant overload puts a strain on this system.

Eating Prudently

There is an old story about a cowboy who would not eat jerky because he had heard that we are what we eat. In a certain sense, the cowboy was right; our body is in trouble if we do not feed it what it needs, or if it cannot handle (metabolize) what we feed it. Eating "healthy" foods should indeed make us healthy; eating "unhealthy" foods may rob us of our health. On the other hand, everything we eat is treated by our digestive tract in the same impersonal way, broken down completely into its building blocks (starches to glucose, proteins to amino acids, triglycerides into fatty acids), be it a piece of cake or a brussels sprout.

A common belief persisted until recently that people develop diabetes from eating too much refined sugar. The most recent studies do not support this belief.

Furthermore, people in countries that consume a lot of carbohydrates in the form of pasta or rice do not have a higher frequency of diabetes than do people in countries where larger amounts of protein and fat are eaten. Therefore, it seems that the primary enemy is not so much *what* we eat as *how much* we eat (coupled with subsequent development of obesity).

Once a person becomes diabetic, however, he or she cannot eat with impunity. Then, the kinds of sugars and carbohydrates consumed do indeed make a difference. The basic proportions of carbohydrate, protein, and fat should ideally be the same for a diabetic and a nondiabetic. Still, the diabetic *cannot* eat those sugars—glucose and sucrose—that are rapidly absorbed, because insulin cannot be released fast enough from the pancreas (in the Type II diabetic) or from the site of an injection (in the Type I diabetic) to handle them. A recommended diet consists of approximately 55 percent carbohydrates, 20 percent proteins, and 30 percent fats.

The Viruses

Information available from human studies regarding the types of viruses that cause diabetes is still very limited. But on the basis of animal studies, it would seem that there are several viruses with the potential to cause diabetes in humans.

One recent study involved a child who died shortly after the onset of Type I diabetes. Researchers extracted a coxsackie B-4 type virus from the child's pancreas. When mice were then inoculated with this virus, they also developed a full-blown syndrome of Type I diabetes. Subsequently, the coxsackie B-4 type virus was recovered from their pancreases as well, indicating to researchers that the virus was certainly instrumental in the destruction of the beta cells and hence probably caused diabetes in both the child and the mice. (While a number of other viruses are suspected of causing diabetes, the evidence is not clear cut.)

It would seem, however, that the virus alone is not to blame. The virus is only part of the problem. Apparently, antigens on the surface of the virus are similar to antigens on the beta cells—so the immune cells or antibodies we produce to destroy the virus may also attack our own cells. Therefore, it is not only the virus that kills the beta cells; it is our own immune system as well.

You may wonder why the neighboring alpha cells are not also destroyed. The answer is that the alpha cells do not have the same antigens on their surface as the beta cells do, so the antibodies and immune cells do not attack them. Every antigen has its own specific binding site, which the corresponding antibodies and immune cells recognize; the antibodies can cling onto and attack *only* their designated antigens.

Diabetes Caused by Poisons

There are a number of chemical agents that will selectively destroy beta cells. Some are widely used for producing experimental diabetes in animals. Also, there are documented cases in which people who survived after eating certain kinds of rat poison suffered the destruction of their beta cells and hence became diabetic. It is of interest that those people who have no diabetic relatives developed changes in their blood vessels identical to those in diabetics who are genetically predisposed to diabetes.

But such poisons are rarely the cause of diabetes in humans. The main enemy we face is, ironically, one over which we do have control—if we choose to exercise it. That enemy is our tendency, because we live in a prosperous culture, to overeat and let ourselves get fat.

CHAPTER 7

How We Get Fat . . . How We Get Thin

"Let me have men about me that are fat; sleek-headed men, and such as sleep o' nights. Yon Cassius has a lean and hungry look; he thinks too much: such men are dangerous." Those are the words of Shakespeare's Julius Caesar, who seems to be implying that fat men are not as conniving as thin men, or, perhaps, do not possess the same energy for mischief. And there is little argument about the implications of the second part. Extra bulk certainly puts a strain on a person's ability to move as fast as he did when he was thinner.

So how does one think thin? How does one get thin? Perhaps, more important, why does one get fat? Once we know that, perhaps we can work on preventive procedures for ourselves, or figure out a healthy way to reverse the process and lose weight.

To begin with, we must be careful not to listen to certain so-called diet experts who are nothing but doomsayers. Some of these individuals have authoritative voices, but they lack complete knowledge of the body's cellular structures and their functions. For instance, one such "expert" regularly states that as a person gets fat, more fat cells develop, and that then, when a person diets, those extra fat cells will not go away but will forever secrete an enzyme that creates in the once-obese individual the nagging desire to eat until those fat cells are once again filled. Obviously, his description of the Curse of Fat is something on a par with being bitten by a werewolf.

Before we can take a logical approach to diet—one that is immune to superstition and pessimistic heresay—it is necessary to understand how our metabolism responds to various influences (both physiological and psychological). We can start by understanding just how those fat cells *do* behave.

How Our Fat Cells Work

The total number of fat cells in any one person can increase in number during early childhood. After that time, however, they probably do not increase in number to any significant extent. They do, however, increase in size.

Conversely, fat cells do not decrease in number either; they will, however, decrease in size. (But there is no evidence that any enzyme is secreted from the fat cells of a dieting person to produce hunger.) When the cell starts losing fat, it shrinks.

Our bodies consist of complex systems, and medical science is still struggling to understand the relationships between those systems. What makes us hungry is not the fat cells crying out to be satiated, but the hypothalamus, which is at the base of the brain. That we know. What we don't know is why.

Regulators of Appetite and Metabolism

We know that if a specific area in the hypothalamus is damaged, obesity can result (in humans as well as in laboratory mice). This problem is most often seen in children with pituitary tumors.

The pituitary gland is situated right next to the hypothalamus. When the tumor enlarges and presses on the hypothalamus, the appetite may be overstimulated; the children in whom this occurs are driven to overeat and hence become enormously fat.

The thyroid gland, which greatly influences metabolism, also affects body weight. The thyroid gland is situated in the neck and secretes a hormone called thyroxine, which regulates our "thermostats" by controlling the rate at which we metabolize (or "burn") what we eat. And the thyroid can be chemically stimulated or suppressed to increase or decrease its thyroxine output (though stimulating a normally functioning thyroid just to "get thin" is never a good idea).

People who have an innately underactive thyroid (hypothyroidism) do not produce enough thyroxine and may gain weight as a result of a sluggish metabolism and water retention; thyroxine supplements prescribed by a doctor can quickly help remedy the problem. Conversely, those who suffer from hyperthyroidism (an overactive thyroid gland) experience the unpleasant side effects of an abnormally sped-up metabolism. Again, prescribed medication can bring the metabolism back to normal.

Doctors generally keep an eye on a patient's thyroid function through routine checkups and blood tests, since thyroxine output can change during the course of one's life.

Pondering the Effects of Aging

One popular notion which has yet to be proved is that a person's metabolism changes—slows down—as he or she gets older.

One thing that most certainly does happen as people get older is that their physical activity tends to decrease. However, it is hard to know what is cart and what is horse here. We do know that the less exercise a person gets, the fewer calories are burned. The question is, *why* is the person less physically active? Is it because enzymatic machinery loses efficiency, making it increasingly difficult for the individual's body to burn the fuel to produce the energy necessary for physical activity? Or is it something else? Could the reasons be more psychological than physiological? We don't know yet—though we do know, for instance, that some overeating is rooted in purely psychological causes. When it comes to understanding the relationship between metabolism and aging, we're still making educated guesses, which are not the same as scientific demonstrations. It is clear that the older person requires fewer calories to maintain his or her weight because physical activity and daily caloric expenditure is decreased.

Stress

People do burn calories by thinking, but not very many. Stress, however, can burn up a lot of calories through what is commonly called "nervous energy." Many of the hormones released under conditions of stress promote the breakdown and burning of fat. Under these circumstances, someone who was skinny all through school because of stressful competition might gain weight when he or she gets out of school simply because he or she continues to eat as though still under stress.

The hormone released in response to stress is adrenaline, the same one that's released when you are frightened, or running, or nervous about having to speak in front of an audience. So if you're under stress all the time, production of this hormone is high all the time, too. When that happens, your muscles are "turned on"; you simply can't sit still.

If under these stressful circumstances your metabolism is flooding the body with energy that has to be expended somehow—such as running from danger or constantly fidgeting—metabolism would appear to be governing physical activity. That, however, is currently a lot harder to prove than that physical activity increases metabolism. The point is that stress leads to increased physical activity (nervous energy), which leads to an increase in calorie burning. During times of stress, energy stores are metabolized faster than at times of, say, rest or leisure activity. (We will explore the effects of stress on the diabetic more thoroughly in Chapter 16.)

How Our Bodies React to Fasting

Some of the so-called diet experts are advocates of fasting as a way to hasten weight loss—that is, consuming nothing but water and skipping meals entirely. Before you're tempted by this approach, you should know that the effects of complete fasting on the human body have been extensively studied, and the findings show that fasting is physically *harmful.* We mentioned these ill effects in Chapter 4, but they cannot be stressed enough.

Why can't a person maintain a healthy body while ingesting only water? When you eat no food and drink just water, your body's stored fat is broken down into fatty acids and used without modification as fuel by many cells. However, other cells, including those of the brain, require most of their fuel in the form of glucose. To obtain glucose when there is no ready food, amino acids released from muscle cells go to the liver and are turned into glucose there. This process, as we've said, reduces the availability of these amino acids for re-use by muscle cells (meanwhile, the muscle cells are probably losing bulk as a result of drastically reduced exercise). Extended total fasting can also create a salt-to-water imbalance, which can upset the cardiovascular system and even cause sudden death.

On a partial fast (or balanced diet), it takes a person a little longer to lose weight and get rid of fat than on a total fast, but the muscles are spared. Furthermore, this person will have more strength and be in a better all-around state of physical and mental health.

Changing Your Eating Habits

A person trying to lose weight needs to stick to a balanced diet that reduces and perhaps redistributes the number of calories consumed. The long-term success of any diet generally requires a permanent reduction in the amount of food consumed.

It is obviously far more appealing to people to undertake a temporary diet program, one that has an end in sight, after which they can return to old eating habits. Many people can discipline themselves for a short time, but knowing that they must eat less for the rest of their lives is much harder to accept. (Actually, once an individual has achieved the desired weight loss on a balanced diet, he or she may be able to increase food consumption somewhat, to maintain that weight.) The person who can lose weight gradually by developing better eating habits through actual behavior modification is much more likely to be able to maintain the weight loss than someone who uses short-term or fad diets to reduce.

Special Concerns for the Overweight Diabetic

As we've said before, a fat person has a better chance of becoming diabetic than a thin person. To summarize our previous discussions, the current hypothesis is that as a person becomes fat, he or she has a larger mass of tissue requiring insulin. The pancreas does not make more beta cells to accommodate this mass, so it is placed under a strain. At the same time that the fat cells are growing larger, there is a reduction in the insulin receptors on the surface of those cells.

This reduction in receptors contributes to the condition known as *insulin resistance;* it takes more insulin than usual to do the job, since there are fewer receptors per cell. This puts even further strain on the pancreas. Presumably, then, the reason people become diabetic is that their need for insulin exceeds their pancreatic reserve and, therefore, the ability of the insulin to maintain normal blood sugar.

Fortunately, when some of these people lose weight—and often it does not take very much of a weight loss—they reduce their insulin resistance, and consequently reduce the demand on their pancreatic reserve. Because the body mass is reduced and enough receptors are back in place to do their job (how those receptors replenish themselves is not yet known), blood sugar levels return to normal.

It seems, however, that some people experience a gradual loss of pancreatic reserve throughout their lives, independent of weight loss or gain. Such an individual might have to lose more weight than another would, or modify the content of his or her diet to correct the diabetes. Or perhaps this individual would have to lose more weight at a given age than he or she would have had to lose earlier, when the reserve was larger.

CHAPTER 8

Diabetes in Women

It is widely believed that there are more female than male diabetics, but numbers can be deceptive. Since 40 percent of the diabetic population is over the age of sixty-five, and since women generally outlive men, it stands to reason that women have a greater risk of developing diabetes just because more of them live longer.

In addition, women in general are not as physically active as men. As they reach middle age, they have a greater tendency to put on weight. And as has been established, fat people are more in danger of becoming diabetic than thin people are. Since obesity is a factor in insulin resistance, and since it is known that women have more fat per body mass than men, they tend to become insulin resistant more quickly than men do, eventually risking diabetes.

Beyond that, the increased demands for insulin associated with childbearing may stress insulin reserves and also predispose women to diabetes later in life.

Another factor that might contribute to the apparent high frequency of diabetes in women (and here's where the statistics may be particularly deceiving) is that they tend to see their physicians more frequently than men do. This could occur partly because women need to seek a doctor's advice not just for the illnesses common to both sexes but for menstrual problems, pregnancy, pap smears, etc. In this case, if a woman is diabetic, she has greater opportunity than a man would to have her disease diagnosed because, as we've said, milder cases of Type II diabetes are often discovered "accidentally" when the doctor does routine tests to explore some unrelated complaint.

Urinary and Vaginal Infections

Diabetic women who are well controlled have little related trouble with menstrual and urogenital disorders. But those who are not well controlled will have noticeably more problems in this area than do nondiabetic women. They are prone to infections, which may necessitate repeated office visits or hospitalizations.

Because of their shorter urethra (the tube carrying urine to the outside from the bladder), women are more susceptible to bladder infections than men are. Sugar in the urine creates a favorable environment for bacteria, increasing the likelihood of infection. This can be a problem especially for an older woman who does not completely empty her bladder. The urine remaining in the bladder constitutes a stagnant pool in which bacterial growth is encouraged by the high glucose levels.

Vaginal infections also can be an extra nuisance for the poorly controlled diabetic. Here again, higher glucose levels make the vagina hospitable to yeast, bacteria, and other infectious organisms.

Sexual Function

It is generally believed that diabetes has relatively little effect on sexual function in women in contrast to men (see Chapter 9). This may be because the major difficulty diabetic men experience is impotence which appears to be basically a problem related to impaired function of the nerves that control blood flow in the penis and, therefore, the ability to achieve an erection. In contrast, the nerves involved in achieving orgasm appear to be much less affected in men as well as in women.

There are relatively few studies of effects of diabetes on a woman's ability to respond to sexual stimulation and enjoy sexual intercourse—and the findings in these studies are not in complete agreement. In one study as many as one-third of diabetic women were reported to be unable to experience climax; in another comparable study, no similar problems were reported.

However, diabetic women who are not in good control may tend to experience more discomfort during intercourse and may be more likely to have bladder and/or vaginal infections related to intercourse because of decreased vaginal secretions. This problem usually can be helped with appropriate lubricants and vaginal creams.

Diabetes and Pregnancy

Since Type II diabetics are generally over forty, most diabetic women going through pregnancy and childbirth are the younger, Type I diabetics. If the diabetic woman of childbearing age is under control, which means that her blood sugar levels are brought down to within the normal range *before conception,* and kept that way throughout her pregnancy, her child will be at almost no greater risk of having congenital malformations than will the child of a nondiabetic woman.

However, it is extremely important that she achieve this control *before* she conceives. As soon as the egg is fertilized and the cells start dividing, the fetus begins to develop. During the period of cell division, the cells undergo differentiation, the process in which specialized organs and tissues are being formed.

It is this process of differentiation that determines more than anything else whether the baby will develop normally.

When the Fetus Is Subjected to High Blood Sugar

All the various steps of differentiation, which take place within the first three months of pregnancy, are very sensitive to potential harm from the environment—from radiation, alcohol consumption, cigarette smoking, and some medications, for example. Consequently, it is important that the child have a normal metabolic environment during the differentiation process.

A poorly controlled diabetic woman usually has no trouble becoming pregnant. The difficulty lies in having a healthy, live baby. If poorly controlled, she will run a greater-than-normal risk of complications including miscarriage, infant death at birth, infant sickness immediately after birth, and congenital defects.

Once the first three months have passed and the differentiation process has been completed, high blood sugar will not affect the developmental process as much as it will create problems related to hormonal and metabolic imbalances. High blood sugar can cause the baby to be overfed and to retain fluids so that it becomes overweight, which may make delivery difficult.

If a baby is subjected to a high maternal blood sugar level, its pancreas will produce insulin to bring its own body's glucose level into the normal range. In effect, the baby's pancreas overproduces insulin in order to utilize the excess glucose being supplied by the mother. However, at delivery, when the cord is cut, the baby's pancreas cannot shut off the production of insulin quickly enough. As a result, since the insulin is still compensating for a glucose supply that's been cut off, the baby can quickly become hypoglycemic, a condition that can cause brain damage. The brain must have glucose, and the excessive insulin level can lower the blood glucose level enough to deprive the brain of what it needs. Today's obstetricians and pediatricians are aware of this potential problem and closely monitor the baby's blood sugar.

Underdeveloped Big Babies

The big babies produced by poorly controlled diabetic women and the excessive amniotic fluid that these women carry in their uteruses combine to make a diabetic woman a leading candidate for cesarean delivery. Today, well-controlled diabetic mothers are able to carry the child to full term or to near full term because of better management. Being able to carry the child to full term decreases the risk of the baby having lung maturation problems. It may seem incredible, but an 11- or a 12-pound baby may have lungs that have not developed enough to sustain it.

These problems highlight the importance of good prenatal care. In addition, it is more critical that the baby of a diabetic woman be born in a hospital where a doctor can obtain blood test results in minutes and start treatment immediately. Before birth, the doctor can check on the fetus's lung development by taking a sample of the amniotic fluid which will give clues as to whether the lungs are mature. In addition, images obtained from ultrasound waves can be used to get a picture of the baby's size, weight, maturity, and the possible presence of congenital malformations.

The Extra Demand for Insulin during Pregnancy

When the controlled diabetic woman becomes pregnant, she is on a certain insulin dosage. After conception, insulin requirements must be adjusted every few weeks by the physician, and perhaps daily by the woman herself. (She should be on a program of self blood glucose monitoring.) Particularly during the second trimester, the fourth through sixth month of pregnancy, a woman's insulin requirement increases. By the time she gets past the third month, she may have gradually increased her food intake by 500 to 1,000 calories a day. The baby is getting bigger. The woman's heart is pumping more blood. The body is working harder to carry that extra weight and to create new tissue. In addition, metabolic demands on her body are increasing because of the increased caloric intake. As a result, she needs more insulin, perhaps twice as much as she did before she became pregnant.

For the pregnant diabetic, there is a sharply increased danger of ketoacidosis, which once was usually fatal for the mother, though medicine has now made advances in this area. On the other hand, if the mother does develop prolonged ketoacidosis, there still is a high probability—up to 95 percent—that the fetus will die.

During the final trimester, insulin requirements increase yet further. Ketoacidosis is still a risk but is not, at this point in the pregnancy, as potentially lethal to the fetus.

During labor, insulin requirements decrease dramatically. When a woman delivers, the hormones that counteract insulin are expelled with the placenta. So the amount of circulating insulin is not being opposed, and the mother may be able to go three to five days requiring minimal amounts of insulin. However, in a few days she will be back to "normal," taking approximately the same dosage she did before getting pregnant.

Temporary Diabetes during Pregnancy

If a nondiabetic woman develops diabetes during pregnancy (gestational diabetes), it is usually a temporary condition due to the increased demand on her pancreas caused both by hormonal changes and by the increased nutritional intake she requires to support a fetus. The condition must be managed so that the blood sugar is normalized, just as it is for any other diabetic.

And although the condition is likely to disappear after childbirth, it is a warning that the reserves of the pancreas are limited and cannot handle additional stress; the woman must be careful to avoid excess weight gain, or she may develop full-blown diabetes later in life.

It is particularly important before conception and during the first trimester for the diabetic mother to control her blood sugar. As discussed in Chapter 14 ("Determining the Insulin Dosage") a single dose of insulin a day is unlikely to provide good control in the pregnant diabetic. In addition, the diabetic mother who needs insulin and takes only one injection a day is risking miscarriage or a birth defect in her offspring to a much higher extent than the pregnant diabetic who takes two or more shots a day or who uses an insulin pump to control her blood sugar. Her baby will also run a greater risk of being overweight, and hence of developing the hypoglycemia and respiratory problems mentioned earlier.

Insulin taken by injection does not harm the unborn child. The important factor for the child's well being is the mother's degree of control. The baby takes what it needs from the mother.

As we said before, almost all pregnant diabetic women are Type I. But those who are Type II, even if their abnormality is mild, also should have their blood sugar levels controlled through diet and, if necessary, insulin. Oral agents are not approved for use during pregnancy.

Morning Sickness

Morning sickness can be a major problem for a diabetic woman because of the threat of insulin reaction and ketoacidosis. Remember that the amount of insulin taken is based on the assumption that the person is going to consume a certain number of calories for breakfast, lunch, dinner, and snacks at approximately the same time each day. If the person is unable to eat or drink, and if she has taken her insulin, she is susceptible to insulin reaction. On the other hand, if not enough insulin is taken, the blood sugar is going to rise.

This is one of the Catch-22s of medicine, kind of a darned-if-you-do and darned-if-you-don't situation. One of the things that many diabetics do not realize is that their liver continues to produce glucose even if they do not eat. Diabetics may rationalize that if they do not eat, then they don't need to take insulin because their blood sugar cannot be high. It just doesn't work that way. In the absence of insulin, the liver continues to make glucose from amino acids formed from muscle breakdown. Therefore, it is important to check the urine for sugar and ketones and use self blood glucose monitoring measurements to determine the amount of insulin to take.

Susceptibility of Offspring

A question that many pregnant diabetics ask their doctor is, "Will my child be diabetic?" Susceptibility to diabetes *is* passed along through the genes (from either parent). But a recent study at the University of Pittsburgh indicated that only 2–3 percent of children with one diabetic parent develop the disease. If a sibling, as well as one parent, is diabetic, the chances of a child developing diabetes increases to about 12 percent. If neither parent is diabetic, but they have one diabetic child, the chance of any of their other children developing diabetes is about 6–7 percent.

Susceptibility to Heart Disease

Diabetes makes women equal to men in their susceptibility to heart disease. That means diabetic women develop heart disease and cardiovascular complications at a younger age than do nondiabetic women. Why this happens is not entirely clear. It may be due to alterations in the balance of hormones. It is known that the increased incidence of cigarette smoking among all women, diabetic and nondiabetic, has increased their incidence of heart disease and cardiovascular problems.

Joys of Life

The female diabetic *who is properly educated* about her disease, and *who is able to achieve reasonably good control,* should be able to live a relatively normal life span with minimal or delayed complications. She can get married, become pregnant, have children, and look forward to most of the pleasures and rewards that a nondiabetic woman enjoys.

CHAPTER 9

. . . And in Men

Sexual Function

The male diabetic, like the female diabetic, has problems that are uniquely his own. Prominent among these potential problems is impotence—the inability to generate and maintain an erection.

Even in a man who is functional in every other respect, deprivation of sexual activity may cripple his sense of well-being and his daily interaction with other people. If he can no longer function sexually, he may feel severely inadequate and depressed. In such an individual, a successful penile implant may be as important to his general health and well-being as efforts to normalize his blood glucose and maintain a balanced diet.

An erection is a remarkable physical phenomenon. In the anticipation of sexual activity, the vein carrying blood from the penis constricts. Arterial flow then allows for vascular engorgement, making the penis erect and hard. If a man is physically unable to generate an erection, something has clearly happened to prevent constriction; the blood flowing into the penis is flowing right back out again.

Nerve Damage

Since the constriction of the vein draining the penis is controlled by the nervous system, the general belief among medical experts is that impotence caused by diabetes is the result of nerve damage, technically known as neuropathy.

However, there may be more to the problem than that. Research focusing on the responses of the blood vessels to chemicals that normally make them constrict or dilate has demonstrated that such responses are altered in diabetics. Those studies suggest that in certain cases of impotence, nerves to the vein draining the blood from the penis may be normal but the vein itself is simply not responding to neural or hormonal stimulation. Some of these changes appear to occur long before there is any evidence of neuropathy in the diabetic. Still another potential cause is narrowing of the artery that supplies blood to the penis (as a consequence of other vascular diseases).

Still other research suggests that in diabetics there are also early changes in the smooth muscles cells, which control ejaculation. This results in the inability to ejaculate, another type of impotence.

Until further research has been completed, the question of what causes impotence in diabetics is open for debate, as is the question of whether the condition is reversible. Most likely it will turn out that, in the diabetic as well as in the nondiabetic, impotence may be caused by several different conditions. If the cause does prove to be damaged nerves, the prospect for cure is probably not very good. Some experts, however, feel that in a young diabetic such damage might be reversible. However, it stands to reason—with the knowledge presently available to us—that if the damage is extensive, the resulting impotence is permanent.

In general, men suffer from impotence for a wide variety of reasons. Ten to fifteen years ago, physicians thought that 90 percent of impotence was due to psychological causes. Now that thinking has reversed, and it is believed that only 10 percent is psychologically rooted, with the greater percentage attributed to organic problems. Most impotent men are diabetics.

Other organic disturbances known to precipitate impotence include multiple sclerosis, cancers of the bladder and bowels, and traumatic injury, as well as radical pelvic surgery and removal of the prostate gland. A number of medications used to treat high blood pressure, heart disease, and depression also may cause impotence, though the problem usually disappears when medication is withdrawn.

The Use of Penile Implants

But even men who face permanent impotence—for whatever reason—do not have to see their sex life end. The development of penile prosthesis implants has been a great help to such men, many of them diabetics. Patients who have successful implants are no longer rare, but because of the "delicacy" of the subject, the public doesn't get much exposure to information about this helpful treatment.

The first surgical implants were accomplished in the late 1950s. They were not cosmetically pleasing, and sometimes there were medical complications. Modern-day prostheses, however, cause less tissue reaction and less scar formation. Consequently, the body is less likely to "reject" the implant.

There are two major types of implants currently in use. One is an inflatable prosthesis that was developed in the early 1970s by F. B. Scott, an American urologist. The Scott prosthesis is a hydraulic system of dacron-reinforced silicone rubber. Under the lower abdominal muscles near the groin, a reservoir is placed to hold the fluid that is used to activate the device. Two pumps placed in the scrotum are used for inflating and deflating the prosthesis once it has been surgically inserted into the penis. The pumps are bulblike devices that are simply squeezed manually to transfer the fluid in their reservoirs to the tubes in the penis. The prosthesis itself consists of two cylinders connected by tubing to the remainder of the system.

The other type of prosthesis—developed recently in Germany—is a malleable silicone cylinder surrounding woven silver wire. It is not an inflatable device, but can be bent upwards for intercourse as the silver wire provides the required rigidity.

How Well Do They Work? Sensation and satisfaction for the recipients depend on several factors, including the extent of neuropathy and the enjoyment the man derives from being able simply to engage in sexual activity and to please his partner. Of the models currently available, most men appear to prefer the inflatable prostheses.

Generally speaking, the implants have no effect on the ability of the recipient to climax. Indeed, the majority of impotent diabetic men are still able to climax. The implants simply provide an erection which makes sexual intercourse possible. In this regard, we should point out that there are actually two types of impotence. The one we have been discussing is erectile impotence. This is the type which benefits by a penile prosthesis. The other type of impotence, mentioned earlier, is the inability to ejaculate. This form is usually unaffected by penile prosthesis.

One urologist stated that approximately 35 percent of all patients who receive penile prostheses are diabetics. The average age for those receiving the implants is between 55 and 65. One of the reasons this age range is so high, he says, is that impotent men frequently will wait several years before seeking advice.

Men are reluctant to seek advice on the problem of impotence for many reasons, not the least of which is ignorance as to the cause of the problem. They may think the problem is hopeless or that it's caused by job-related anxiety, or they may be having marital problems and assume that's the source of trouble. Sometimes they are just not interested, because no partner is involved.

Worse, perhaps, is the situation in which a patient's doctor is not sympathetic to the problem, or not concerned enough to pursue it, assuming that a man of his age—say, fifty-five—is not interested in sex. If you are a diabetic male with an impotence problem, you should see a urologist who is *experienced in the use of penile prostheses* to find out if you would benefit from such a device.

Reproductive Concerns

Another question that may arise concerns the effect of diabetes on the viability and health of the sperm (i.e., will the sperm from a diabetic man produce a healthy baby?). The answer to that—like the answers to many questions involving diabetes—is not clearly established. However, most of the evidence available indicates that it is not a defect in the sperm or the egg that causes defects in an embryo but, rather, the environment of the uterus in which the embryo develops and grows during the first trimester of pregnancy.

Susceptibility to diabetes is passed along through the genes of either parent. See Chapter 8, under "Diabetes and Pregnancy" for more information.

PART TWO

The Research and the Controversies

CHAPTER 10

What We Know So Far

Today, we are able to write about the facts behind diabetes as if they were obvious truths, as if they have been common knowledge for centuries. However, such appearances are deceiving. The learning process has been painfully slow, involving long periods of research punctuated by brief, transient moments of glorious discovery. And even now, medical experts argue over some of the broadest issues surrounding diabetes and its treatment.

It was only in the 1860s that the German medical student, Paul Langerhans, discovered the presence of clusters of cells in the pancreas that were different from the rest of the tissue in the gland.

Decades passed, however, before researchers figured out that the islets had something to do with sugar metabolism. Many more years elapsed before, in the early 1900s, a series of studies by several different investigators revealed that in animals the islets were secreting a substance into the blood which prevented diabetes. That substance was named *insulin* (from the Latin word for island) because of its close relationship to the Islets of Langerhans.

The First Effective Diabetes Treatment

Finally, in 1921, Frederick G. Banting, a Canadian physician, with the help of Charles H. Best, a medical student, extracted insulin from the pancreas for the first time. At last medical science had found an effective way to treat insulin-dependent diabetes. Banting achieved this feat when he was only twenty-nine years old. It earned him a Nobel Prize and knighthood.

That initial extraction came on the heels of a long line of experiments based on a series of ideas from many investigators. Banting's idea for the possible extraction had been suggested by something he had read in a surgical journal. If you were to block the pancreatic duct, he reasoned, that might cause destruction of the exocrine cells (those that secrete digestive enzymes into the intestine through the duct). The islets are not connected to the duct; they secrete their products (insulin and glucagon) directly into the bloodstream. Therefore, Banting reasoned, if you could destroy the exocrine cells by blocking the pancreatic duct, you'd be left with the endocrine (islet) cells intact; and if the islets were not destroyed, what you'd extract from the pancreas would be almost pure hormones—which indeed turned out to be the case.

After following the above procedure, Banting and Best managed to extract insulin from the pancreas of a dog. They ground up the pancreas and injected some of the extracted solution into another dog that had fallen into a diabetic coma. Within two hours the dog was up and around.

In January 1922, the first human received a crude extract of insulin obtained from the pancreatic glands of slaughtered cattle. By 1923, relatively pure insulin solutions were available to the masses. The search then began for ways to further purify and modify the insulin to be used for treatment.

Insulin: Where We Get It

Most insulin being used to treat diabetics today comes from pigs and cattle. Pork insulin is much more like that of humans than insulin from any other species except from primates. The extraction and preparation of this substitute insulin is a long, involved, and costly process. The hormone can be extracted efficiently only under very precise conditions of acidity and alcohol concentration, taking advantage of its solubility in alcohol. The process selectively extracts insulin from the pancreas, leaving behind most other proteins.

You might ask, "If a human can accept a pig's insulin, why can't he accept a pig's pancreas, or at least the Islets of Langerhans?" The answer is that humans can accept many purified proteins from other species, but what determines *which* ones is the similarity of those proteins to human proteins. If a single foreign protein is similar enough to the corresponding human protein, the human body will not recognize it as foreign and hence will not attack and reject it.

Transplants are a whole different ballgame. When you transplant an entire organ, you are dealing with a mass of tissue including many different cell types with numerous surface antigens and different proteins. If the recipient's immune system rejects even one of these antigens or cells, this can trigger rejection of the whole organ. This risk exists even with a transplant from one human being to another. When the organ is from a different species, the chances of rejection are multiplied. As far as the body is concerned, any unfamiliar substances are enemies, and the immune system will produce immune cells and antibodies to destroy them. The reaction that follows may be so severe that the entire organ is destroyed.

When something like insulin is injected into the body, what is being introduced is a single purified protein that is very similar to the corresponding human protein. The body can accept that. (Although many diabetics may make antibodies to injected insulins, the amounts of such antibodies usually do not cause significant problems.)

Refining the Process

Over the years, many advances have been made in modifying synthesized insulins to alter their rate of absorption from the tissues and their availability to the body.

The major emphasis in developing new insulins has not been on creating new *types* so much as on enhancing the purification process itself. Major efforts have been made to eliminate other components that "come with" the extracted insulin (such as the hormone glucagon, from the alpha cells) as well as impurities that may stimulate the production of antibodies.

There is also considerable interest in the production of "human" insulin. One method involves using new recombinant DNA techniques employed in genetic research. This is an exciting development because it could provide an unlimited supply of insulin virtually identical to that made by our bodies. But even this synthesized "human" insulin is not exactly the same as insulin made in the body; the procedures required for preparing and purifying this type of insulin for injection cause subtle structural changes in some of the insulin molecules, making them slightly antigenic. Purified pork insulins are also being chemically modified to produce "human" insulin. When either of these is injected, the slightly altered insulin molecules can cause antibody production similar to that induced by injections of even the most highly purified pork insulin. This is not thought to be a serious problem, however, and many diabetics who are resistant to most purified preparations of animal insulin respond well to synthetic human insulin.

Measuring Our Reserves

Chemically, insulin is a protein molecule made up of 51 amino acids. Scientists have broken it down into its components and even synthesized it in the laboratory. But what do we know about the tiny "factories" that make the insulin, the beta cells? We do know, of course, that the beta cells in some people make and store enough insulin for their metabolic needs, while others don't make nearly enough. So is there any scientific method to find out whether one's beta cells are full, half-full, or nearly empty? In fact, there is.

How Insulin Is Stored

If you look through a microscope at a section of the pancreas, you will see what look like tiny granules in the beta cells. In a normal pancreas, there are lots of these tiny granules, which consist of insulin and are released into the blood on demand.

These granules, the storage form of insulin, are highly concentrated crystals held in tiny membranous sacs. Within these crystals, the insulin is combined with zinc. With the appropriate stimulus, these sacs move to the surface of the beta cell. Then they open and the crystals are released into the extracellular space. The salts in the body fluids outside the cell are very different from those inside and instantly dissolve the insulin. The insulin and zinc then rapidly cross the capillary wall and enter the bloodstream.

Insulin is synthesized in one part of the beta cell and then stored in another part of the same cell until it is needed. It is actually first synthesized as a much larger protein, called pro-insulin. After pro-insulin is formed, a piece splits off. That piece is called C-peptide. What remains is the insulin molecule. Many insulin molecules will clump together with zinc to make a crystal.

In the sac containing the insulin granule, there also will be the waste product, this C-peptide, in the same proportion as insulin. When the cell is stimulated to release its insulin, the waste product is released as well. It is possible to measure the C-peptide level in a sample of blood or urine and thereby to estimate how much insulin a person is able to produce and how much reserve there is.

When There Is a Small Reserve

Some people have a much greater insulin reserve than others. Do such people have extra large beta cells? Probably not. However, their islets of Langerhans may be bigger than average, or they may have more islets or perhaps their islets contain more beta cells. Moreover, their beta cells could make and release insulin at a more efficient rate.

At the opposite extreme, in the case of a Type I diabetic, virtually all the beta cells have been destroyed. But some may still survive and function. Currently, many experts feel that these tiny reserves—if not overworked to the point of exhaustion—could help control blood sugar levels more efficiently than injections alone, since that steady supply, however small, could help offset the fall in blood insulin levels between insulin injections. If even a very small amount of insulin is being produced within the body, it may greatly reduce the risk of ketoacidosis.

Even with a little insulin reserve, the pancreas can usually still respond to a meal in a normal way. It can also respond to increasing blood glucose levels as the last of the injected insulin is wearing off, before the next dose is administered. But to mimic the function of a normal pancreas (with full insulin reserve) as closely as possible, a diabetic with very few remaining beta cells really needs to take boosts of insulin when he eats or at least twice a day. Many physicians think that the development of one-shot-a-day insulin was a mistake and no longer prescribe this method to their patients. It is also very important for the diabetic to be consistent and eat his meals and snacks and take his injections at the same times each day. In addition, the diabetic must learn to coordinate the amount of food and the time at which it is consumed with the timing of injections. This approach seems to be clearly the best means of controlling and managing diabetes.

CHAPTER 11

Controversies about Diabetes

One of the major controversies with respect to diabetes concerns the cause of the complications accompanying the disease. Basically, there are two points of view. One theory attributes the complications to hereditary factors, which, its advocates say, a person inherits *along with* the tendency to become diabetic. The opposing theory attributes the complications directly to the metabolic consequences of an absolute or relative insulin deficiency.

The implication of the first theory is that it does little good to try to normalize blood sugar levels in order to prevent the complications, because the complications are preordained by the person's genes. Followers of this "genetic" theory reason that if there is nothing a physician can do to prevent complications, why waste time trying to normalize blood sugar levels except to prevent ketoacidosis and to alleviate immediate health complaints of the patient? They advocate treating symptoms only and not working to bring the patient's blood sugar as close to normal as possible.

The other point of view holds that those dire complications (e.g., blindness, cardiovascular disease, neuropathy, etc.) are directly caused by chronic, long-term high blood sugar levels and/or the lack of insulin, per se. As you have read in our discussion of the complications in Chapter 5, this is the viewpoint to which we subscribe. Strong evidence supporting this opinion has been mounting over the last several years. As a result, we are confident that if we can restore the metabolic state to normal (normalize blood glucose levels), then we can prevent or markedly delay the onset of complications. Those of us who believe in this principle will make great efforts to work closely with our patients, to educate them, and to try to help them normalize their blood sugar levels.

The Genetic Viewpoint

Proponents of the genetic theory support their viewpoint by citing the high number of cases in which diabetics receiving insulin nevertheless develop complications late in life. They claim that sometimes these complications occur even in diabetics who do not suffer from the symptoms of abnormally high glucose levels.

What that point of view does not recognize, however, is that until the last decade most people who were treated with insulin still had blood sugar levels well above normal much of the time. Not until the early 1970s did physicians appreciate that an individual might have chronic high blood sugar levels that still did not interfere with carrying out daily activities in a relatively normal way, yet which probably were slowly injuring the blood vessels and nerves; this injury eventually causing serious complications. Consequently, although such people may have been getting insulin, it did not prevent the complications *because it was not adequate to normalize their blood sugar levels.*

Since these diabetics seemed to feel all right for a while, their physicians assumed that their bodies were not being harmed. It is on this assumption that advocates of the genetic theory build their case.

To further support their opinion, they cite also those unusual "nondiabetic" individuals with "normal blood sugars" who have been observed to have the complications associated with diabetes. "See?" they say. "It's genetic." But if one investigates further the history of such individuals, it often turns out that they have a history of being overweight and may at those times have actually had undetected diabetes. In any case, as we said in Chapter 5, there is general agreement that the complications of vascular disease *are usually the cause of death* in people with diabetes; what we don't know for certain yet is *how* diabetes causes that vascular injury.

Locating the Source of Damage

The opposing theory supports the idea that the lack of insulin in and of itself could be making the tissues more susceptible to injury, simply because they aren't getting their proper "nourishment" and are hence in a weakened state. Then, too, high blood sugars and other metabolic changes associated with insulin deficiency might be causing additional injury, compounding the problem.

Conversely, it has been suggested that some health problems could arise because diabetics under treatment have *too much* insulin at times. After injection, the level of insulin in the blood is by no means constant. At its peak, that level may be significantly higher than normal. Insulin levels also may be higher than normal between meals in Type II diabetics. These high insulin levels, it has been suggested, might cause problems by increasing cholesterol and lipid formation and accumulation in the walls of the arteries. It should be noted that this theory remains, as yet, unproven.

The Case for High Blood Sugar

But the most significant danger is probably high blood sugar itself. The excess glucose circulating in the blood appears to be damaging or even toxic to susceptible cells. (We described just how that might happen in Chapter 5.)

When this theory was first suggested, it seemed to be the least likely of any of the possible causes for diabetic complications. In fact, if a physician had supported that point of view in the early 1970s, he or she would have been openly laughed at by many colleagues. After all, clinicians could tell you, a person can walk around with blood sugars as high as 600 or 700 milligrams percent and still lead a relatively normal existence. If so, how could high sugar be hurting anything? Diabetics who received supplementary insulin looked okay. They seemed to be getting along reasonably well. The idea that a high glucose level itself could be causing these problems was considered simplistic and naive.

So it came as a great surprise to the medical community when, in the mid-seventies, two adverse effects of excess glucose were discovered. First, researchers showed that relatively large amounts of glucose are converted in some cells to sorbitol, a complex sugar alcohol, which is then trapped inside the cells. The increased rate of formation of this alcohol appears to be responsible for cataracts and nerve damage, among other disorders, and is associated with increased blood flow and vascular leakage in research animals with diabetes.

Since the enzymes that facilitate the conversion of glucose to sorbitol are present in virtually all tissues (including blood vessels), such damage can potentially occur anywhere.

Glycosylation

The second discovery was nonenzymatic glycosylation of proteins (a chemical reaction in which glucose sticks permanently to proteins, even in non-diabetics), including the hemoglobin in the red blood cells. Since the average red cell survives about 120 days, the longer it circulates, the more sugar one will find bound to the hemoglobin in that cell. The term for this process is nonenzymatic glycosylation because no enzyme is involved.

In the nondiabetic, about 5 percent of the hemoglobin is glycosylated at any one time. In a poorly controlled diabetic, that proportion may be as high as 20 percent. Glycosylated hemoglobin does not function properly. For one thing, it does not release oxygen to the tissues as readily as nonglycosylated hemoglobin will. This breakdown in efficiency might contribute to oxygen shortage in an organ such as the eye, which needs a lot of oxygen and is one of the organs most affected by the complications of diabetes. Another potential effect of nonenzymatic glycosylation of vessels is that it may lead to impaired filtration function in the kidney and increased vascular leakage throughout the body as discussed in Chapter 5.

Clearly, such findings have contributed to a more widespread acceptance of normalization of blood glucose levels as a major goal of diabetes therapy.

How We Entered the Fray

Our first involvement in this controversy began in 1968 when Dr. Marvin Siperstein published his research findings in the *Journal of Clinical Investigation.* He concluded that his study indicated that thickening of muscle capillary basement membranes is characteristic of genetic diabetes mellitus and that it is independent of carbohydrate derangements (i.e., hyperglycemia) of diabetes mellitus. Statistically, it was difficult to refute Siperstein's observations.

However, our experience with patients in private practice made it difficult for us (and many other diabetes specialists) to accept that conclusion. Although we felt the problem needed further study, Siperstein's conclusions were widely accepted which made it difficult to obtain funding. That did not discourage us, however, and we proceeded with financial support obtained initially from friends and from interested patients who had benefited from blood sugar control. Later we received other private and corporate support. Because of the need for these funds to continue research, in 1972 we established the Kilo Diabetes & Vascular Research Foundation, a not-for-profit organization dedicated to diabetes and vascular disease research and education.

Siperstein's Evidence

Siperstein used a needle to obtain small samples of muscle from the legs of human subjects. When he looked at the muscle capillaries, he saw that their walls were thickened in virtually all the samples obtained from diabetics. This thickening was evidence of vascular disease.

But Siperstein did not find any relationship between the *duration or severity* of diabetes and *degree* of capillary wall thickening. On the basis of this and other findings in his studies, he concluded that ". . . abnormalities of insulin secretion or of carbohydrate metabolism . . . are unlikely to be the factors responsible for the basement membrane thickening and hence the microangiopathy (small vessel disease) of diabetes mellitus."

We believed that the problem in Siperstein's experiment was that most of the subjects he studied were Type II diabetics. Since a Type II diabetic may well have high blood sugar for years before being diagnosed as diabetic, there is no way to accurately determine the time of onset of diabetes. This could explain why Siperstein was unable to show any relationship between apparent duration of diabetes and thickening of capillary basement membranes.

In any case, Siperstein's findings were widely considered to be evidence supporting the theory that vascular disease in diabetics, like the tendency to develop diabetes (insulin deficiency), is primarily hereditary (genetic) rather than a consequence of insulin deficiency or high blood sugar levels. Although Siperstein's findings and the genetic theory in general were not consistent with much of the existing clinical experience, there was no hard evidence to refute them.

What concerned us most was that Siperstein's findings were making a tremendous impact on the treatment of diabetes.

To begin with, it takes a lot of time and attention on the part of physicians, nurses, and dietitians to educate diabetics and their families to learn to live with this disease. And, frankly, many physicians who do not see many diabetics just don't know enough about the condition to do a good job of treating it. What Siperstein's conclusions did was to take a big burden off these doctors' shoulders. If it is all hereditary, they could now reason, there is really no point in trying to get the diabetic's glucose levels back to normal. For obvious reasons, this theory is immensely appealing to many busy physicians as well as to diabetics who find the disease difficult to understand and maintaining the diet, exercise, and medication balance difficult to manage.

Counter-Findings

We decided to repeat Siperstein's research. We used an electron microscope to examine muscle capillaries just as he had, but we studied Type I diabetics, because in these patients the time interval between the development of insulin deficiency and the onset of symptoms which lead to the diagnosis of diabetes is widely accepted to be much shorter than that for Type II diabetes. Thus the time of onset of Type I diabetes can generally be pinpointed much more accurately than the onset of Type II diabetes. We were able to examine, in our younger subjects, the state of the capillaries relatively early after insulin deficiency and high blood sugar levels had set in.

What we found, comparing the tissue in these subjects to that of patients with a longstanding history of diabetes, was that the onset of diabetes preceded the thickening of vessel walls, suggesting that low insulin or high blood sugar may well be the catalyst for damage to the capillary walls, causing them to become leaky and thickened (Figure 1).

Siperstein's most recent study has now confirmed our findings. This was a very interesting study of a group of South Koreans who apparently attempted suicide by ingesting a rat poison which, it was found, produced diabetes in the survivors (who had no family history of diabetes). After a few years of diabetes, a high percentage of these individuals developed the same changes in their muscle capillaries that occur in diabetics in whom the tendency to develop diabetes (but not vascular complications) is known to be genetically controlled. In addition, they also developed evidence of damage to vessels in the eyes and kidneys. Siperstein concluded that "the findings of the present study provide strong evidence that hyperglycemia, or some other abnormality that occurs in insulinopenic (insulin deficient) states, can itself cause the microvascular changes that occur in patients with diabetes mellitus."

These findings support the position that diabetic vascular complications are not purely hereditary in nature; but it still is possible that hereditary risk factors for vascular disease (present in the general population) such as the tendency for high blood cholesterol levels and high blood pressure may accelerate vascular complications in diabetics.

Patients Who Are Difficult to Control

In the face of such evidence, then, how does the pessimistic attitude of so many diabetologists persist?

One reason is that many diabetics who appear to be reasonably well controlled still develop complications while others who

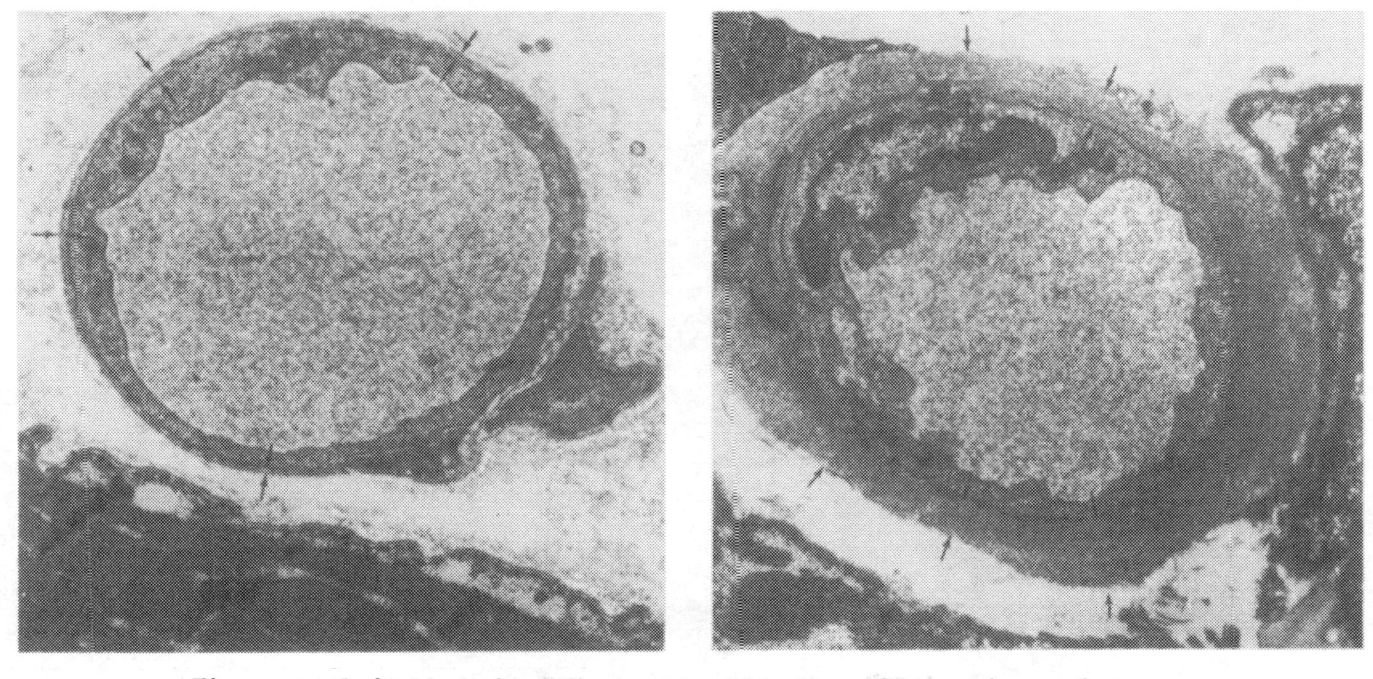

Figure 1 (Left) Normal capillary with a thin basement membrane (between arrows) in the thigh muscle of a nondiabetic person. (Right) A thigh muscle capillary with a very thick basement membrane (between arrows) from a person with poorly controlled diabetes for 15 years.

appear to be poorly controlled have few complications. However, due to the lack of any truly reliable method for accurately assessing overall twenty-four-hour blood glucose levels, it has been impossible to know whether such diabetics were really as well or as poorly controlled as their doctors assumed.

Since blood sugar levels in a diabetic can vary dramatically from one hour to the next, sampling the blood one, two, or even six times a day may not give a reliable estimate of the average level for the day. The same limitation applies to measuring urine sugar.

However, once research showed that excess glucose sticks to the hemoglobin in red blood cells (proportional to blood glucose levels), it became apparent that there might be a successful way to monitor overall sugar levels after all. For instance, since the lifespan of a red cell is about 120 days, a doctor could determine an individual's average sugar level over that time period by measuring the amount of glucose sticking to the patient's red cells. Thus the *glycohemoglobin measurement* is now a way of showing the patient's *average* blood sugar level. For instance, if a patient maintained good control for half the time by keeping the blood sugar at 130 and stayed near 200 the rest of the time, the glycohemoglobin measurement would consistently reflect an average of 165.

New Studies

Numerous recent and ongoing studies are focused on efforts to increase our understanding about how diabetes injures nerves and vessels and on improved treatment to minimize complications in diabetics.

In one such study, conducted at Rockefeller University, a group of diabetics was put on a strict program with the specific aim of bringing down their blood sugar levels.

Throughout the regimen, doctors monitored not only blood sugar, but also glycosylation levels (proportion of glucose sticking to the hemoglobin in the red blood cells), blood platelet function (which, if overstimulated, may contribute to scarring of the vessel walls and hence hardening of the arteries), cholesterol levels, white blood cell function, and blood pressure.

In those patients who were able to normalize their sugars, all of these other functions tended to return to normal, too. Consequently, if all those functions in a diabetic patient were brought to normal—and kept that way through a specific ongoing treatment program—one could predict with reasonable confidence that the risk of cardiovascular disease would decrease sharply. We have conducted similar studies and concluded that blood sugar control will delay or prevent diabetic complications.

Other Experiments

Other investigators are trying to determine whether delivering insulin directly to the liver is more effective than injecting it under the skin. We anticipate some real breakthroughs from some of these investigations. They emphasize the need for studies that can show what in the diabetic state is causing the complications. How much is due to low insulin levels, and how much is due to the subsequent changes such as elevated blood glucose levels that occur because of the insulin deficiency?

The process is long and arduous. Though researchers are anxious to draw hard and fast conclusions, we must all remember what a complicated disease we are dealing with. We must keep in mind, for instance, that diabetes alters the production of numerous hormones—not just insulin. Name a hormone and some researcher has found an effect of diabetes on it. By studying these hormones one at a time, we can hope to unravel a pattern that shows what effects are due to what causes. We need to know, and eventually we will.

References

Feingold, K. R., Lee, T. H., Chung, M. Y., and Siperstein, M. D.: Muscle capillary basement membrane width in patients with vacor-induced diabetes mellitus. *J. Clin. Invest.* 78:102–7, 1986.

Kilo, C., Vogler, N., and Williamson, J. R.: Muscle capillary basement membrane changes related to aging and to diabetes mellitus. Diabetes *21:* 881-905, 1972.

Kilo, C.: Controlling diabetes: should you believe the UGDP? Modern Medicine of Canada 34: 699-704, 1979.

Kilo, C.: The value of glucose control and the measures of control in preventing complications. Am. J. Med. 79 (suppl. 2B): 33-37, 1985.

Rogers, D. G., White, N. H., Santiago, J. V., Miller, P., Weldon, V. W., Kilo, C., and Williamson, J. R.: Glycemic control and bone age are independently associated with muscle capillary basement membrane width in diabetic children after puberty. Diabetes Care *9:* 453-459, 1986.

Siperstein, M. D., Unger, R. H., and Madison, L. L.: Studies of muscle capillary basement membranes in normal subjects, diabetic, and prediabetic patients. *J. Clin. Invest.* 47: 1973-99, 1968.

Sosenko, J. M., Miettinen, O. S., Williamson, J. R. and Gabbay, K. H.: Muscle capillary basement membrane thickness and long-term glycemia in type I diabetes. New Engl. J. Med. *311:* 694-698, 1984.

Williamson, J. R. and Kilo, C.: A common sense approach resolves the basement membrane controversy and the NIH Pima Indian study. Diabetologia *17*: 129-131, 1979.

Williamson, J. R. and Kilo, C.: New evidence that controlling the hyperglycemia of diabetes is important. Resident and Staff Physician April: 46-52, 1979.

CHAPTER 12

Another Setback

Yet another fierce controversy erupted in the early 1970s as the result of a large-scale study conducted by dozens of reputable researchers all over the country. The aim of the project, known collectively as the University Group Diabetes Program (UGDP) was to find out whether insulin treatment and oral medication could prevent the late complications of diabetes. The program began in the early 1960s and involved twelve of the United States' most prestigious medical centers. One of us (Kilo) was involved in the investigation at Washington University in St. Louis.*

Over a period of 8–14 years, more than a thousand newly diagnosed Type II diabetic patients were studied to determine the effectiveness of medical treatment on their disease and its complications. Each institution sent its findings to the same computer center, which then tabulated the results. Before the study was concluded, about $15 million had been spent.

*Dr. Kilo was one of the co-principal UGDP investigators at Washington University and a member of the UGDP executive committee. Once the results of the UGDP study were published, Dr. Williamson joined with Dr. Kilo in analyzing—and refuting—the results.

The patients were divided into five basic care groups: two insulin groups, one in which standardized amounts of insulin were given based on the person's body surface area, and another in which the amount was matched to the patient's individual needs; two groups taking oral agents, one on tolbutamide and the other on phenformin; and an untreated control group for comparison with the other groups given a placebo (a harmless substance substituted for an active medication), plus dietary management. They were all on a diabetic diet designed to achieve desirable body weight.

When the UGDP results were finally reported, one vital conclusion was that "neither insulin nor oral hypoglycemic agents gave better protection against . . . cardiovascular complications of adult-onset diabetes . . . than diet alone." Worse yet, oral agents were not only considered ineffective in lowering blood glucose levels but were suspected of increasing the risk of fatal heart attacks. In addition, the UGDP investigators concluded that "the findings provide no evidence that insulin or any other drug lowering blood glucose levels will alter the course of vascular complications in the type of diabetes that is most common, adult-onset diabetes." (Adult-onset is Type II diabetes.)

The Reaction

The news hit like a bomb. Many of us concerned with the treatment of Type II diabetics knew that insulin and oral agents were indeed effective in controlling blood glucose levels in properly selected and managed patients. Many physicians had been certain that oral agents were effective and safe in appropriate cases, but now felt that if they continued to prescribe them, they might face malpractice suits because of the alleged link to heart attacks.

We and many other researchers were particularly alarmed by these conclusions because they were so different from our own clinical and laboratory experience. And because these conclusions discouraged efforts to normalize blood glucose with insulin and oral agents, we knew that this would result in poorer, rather than improved, treatment of diabetics. Therefore, just as we had done with Siperstein's findings, we undertook a reevaluation of the UGDP data.

Challenging the Computer

Initially, the problem we faced (along with a number of other investigators who wished to examine the UGDP data) was that the computer center would not release the raw data for reevaluation. The officials responsible said the information belonged to each of the respective medical centers that had supplied the data. The Committee for the Care of the Diabetic (a national organization of diabetes specialists) then filed a federal court suit for the release of the data. Eventually the United States Supreme Court concluded that the material belonged to the federal government, so we (and others) were finally able to get a look at it.

The UGDP data was awesome in its sheer volume, and we were at first a bit perplexed as to how we should go about reexamining it. When you have a tremendous amount of data, the tendency is to rely heavily on the computer and to look at computer summaries rather than at individual patient data. As we reflected on what to do, we realized we had to look at the individuals who had died to find out what had gone wrong. What were the circumstances under which each individual died? Were his blood sugars well controlled? Was he taking his assigned medication properly? If you do not study each case individually in this way, you can easily be misled by statistical summaries.

Sleuthing for Flaws

We decided that out of the more than one thousand patients studied, the two hundred people who had died were the bottom line. They were the important people, far more so than those who had survived. To give individual attention to one thousand people is mind-boggling; even examining two hundred in some detail is a major undertaking. We knew, however, that careful scrutiny was essential to understanding the biological significance and meaning of the data.

When we looked closely at the reasons and circumstances of the deaths of those two hundred diabetics, many problems in the computer analysis and conclusions became apparent.

However, what bothered us most was the attitude of many physicians and statisticians toward the UGDP findings—their blind faith in the theory of design of clinical trials, statistical technology, and computer analysis. They seemed to believe that if you design a study very carefully, then nothing serious can go wrong. But, as we all know, that is far from true. To begin with, there are several ways of looking at any one batch of data. If you analyze it in different ways and get the same answers each time, you can be fairly confident of the results and conclusions based on them. If you get conflicting answers, then you know you must search more critically to understand the basis for the discrepancies. That is what we did.

One of the problems with the UGDP as a whole was that a lot of patients involved in the study either dropped out or stopped taking their medication. This behavior is called noncompliance. If the researchers do not look very carefully at the effects of patient noncompliance on results, they can be misled in their interpretations. When we examined the circumstances under which these people died, we found that some of those whose deaths were blamed on the oral agents had in fact not taken those medications for long, because they had dropped out of the group early on. Others, who had been assigned to one of the insulin groups, dropped out and hence did not take the insulin, yet their deaths were counted as part of the data supporting the conclusion that insulin was not beneficial.

We discovered another major problem when we looked at the frequency of heart disease in the control group—those who took the placebo and were managed on diet alone. What initially aroused our suspicion was that the results were not consistent with well-known facts about heart disease in the general diabetic population. For instance, heart disease in the general *nondiabetic* population is a much more serious problem in men than it is in women. Heart attacks are three to four times as common in men, at least until the age when women have passed menopause. In the general *diabetic* population, women lose this advantage; diabetic women are just as likely to die of heart disease as are diabetic men. This statistic has been thoroughly established in many studies.

Yet when we looked critically at the UGDP data, we found that in the placebo diabetic group, the ratio of men to women dying of heart disease was the same as in the nondiabetic population. This indicated that the placebo group was not typical of diabetics in general. Thus the validity of any conclusions based on comparison with this placebo group was, in our opinion, suspect. Contrary to what the official results implied, we found that the untreated diabetics given the placebo had, proportionately, four times the number of heart attacks and strokes as the diabetics treated with insulin doses matched to their individual needs.

Tolbutamide and Phenformin. Tolbutamide and phenformin were the oral agents used in the study which concluded that there was evidence that both drugs produced adverse (harmful) effects on the cardiovascular system.

It is generally acknowledged that if, under a certain prescribed medication, a patient's fasting blood sugar levels cannot be kept below 150–170 mg/dl, he or she should be switched to another medication (i.e., a different oral agent or insulin). What we found was that the apparently greater-than-normal frequency of cardiovascular deaths in the tolbutamide-treated patients could be accounted for by patients whose fasting blood sugars had chronically exceeded 200 yet who had not been switched to another medication! Had these patients not been in a controlled study, presumably (in our opinion) they would have been managed differently. According to our analysis of the data, both tolbutamide and phenformin were safe and effective when used in accordance with conventional guidelines and where patients were compliant in taking their medication as assigned.

A Necessary Reeducation

For more than a decade we and many other diabetes researchers have been trying to clear up the confusion caused by the conclusions published by the UGDP investigators. With all our information available and most of it published in medical journals, it would seem that the controversy should be settled. Fortunately, the American Medical Association and the American Diabetes Association no longer support the results of the UGDP.

However, the controversy lingers on. Surveys taken a few years ago indicate that one out of every three physicians in this country continues to believe (because of the widely publicized UGDP results) that the pills used to lower blood sugar are not safe or effective,* and that blood sugar control is not important in reducing or preventing blood vessel disease.

Because of that decade during which medical schools were teaching the results of the UGDP study, physicians now have to be reeducated through diabetes postgraduate educational programs about what medications are available and how they can

*Perhaps they are not aware that—credibility of the UGDP results aside—many pharmaceutical firms have developed even more effective drugs since the early seventies. These drugs are stronger than the ones we had available to us in the past, yet have fewer side effects. They have been widely used in Europe for more than a decade and were approved by the FDA, in 1984, for use in the United States.

benefit Type II diabetics. Unfortunately, some may not be reached or convinced.

References

Knatterud, G. L., Klimt, C. R., Levin, M. E., Jacobson, M. E., and Goldner, M. G.: Effects of hypoglycemic agents on vascular complications in patients with adult-onset diabetes. VII. Mortality and selected nonfatal events with insulin treatment. *JAMA* 240:37–42, 1978.

Goldner, M. G., Knatterud, G. L., and Prout, T. E.: Effects of hypoglycemic agents on vascular complications in patients with adult-onset diabetes. III. Clinical implications of UGDP results. *JAMA* 218:1400–10, 1971.

Kilo, C. and Williamson, J. R.: Clinical considerations concerning the use of oral antidiabetic agents. In: *Special Topics in Endocrinology and Metabolism. Vol.* 2. (New York: A. R. Liss Inc., 1981) pp. 85–101.

Kilo, C., Miller, J. P., and Williamson, J. R.: The crux of the UGDP. Spurious results and biologically inappropriate data analysis. *Diabetologia* 18:179–85, 1980.

Kilo, C., Miller, J. P., and Williamson, J. R.: The Achilles heel of the University Group Diabetes Program. *JAMA* 243: 450–57, 1980.

PART THREE

The Treatment

CHAPTER 13

Education: An Essential Ingredient

Before Banting and Best isolated the hormone insulin, some of the treatments for diabetes (semi-starvation) were so severe that it is difficult to believe that doctors were prescribing them in the twentieth century. We are fortunate that today medical science has a much better understanding of the human body. The more we know about how the body works, the better we are at correcting malfunctions.

In spite of the mountain of facts indicating that insulin deficiency and the resulting high blood glucose lead to all the complications discussed in Chapter 5, not everyone is convinced that the main goal in the treatment of diabetes should be the normalization of blood glucose. Since we are convinced, we direct our treatment toward that end. In this chapter and the next, we will lay out the basic plan we follow. It involves two basic simultaneous strategies:

1. The establishment of a health program to normalize blood glucose levels.

2. The education and informative counseling of diabetics and their families.

Although we begin both strategies at once, the second is truly the foundation supporting the first, so we will begin by discussing just how we go about accomplishing it. Then, in Chapter 14, we will lay down our guidelines for the practical details of day-to-day management.

The First Concerns

As we mentioned in the very beginning of this book, the first concern a physician usually faces in the treatment of a diabetic is getting the patient to recognize that he or she *does have diabetes,* that it is a *chronic disease,* and that *a person can live with it.* It is natural to deny the disease; but you must get beyond that stage before you can begin to learn what it means for you. Then you must appreciate that it is important to adapt your lifestyle in order to maintain your health and avoid complications. Then the education begins.

If the diabetes is secondary (i.e., a complication of another disease), the physician has a twofold job, which is to correct the primary problem *and* to manage the diabetes. In some instances, when the primary problem is corrected, the diabetes subsides. The patient must know, however, that it makes no difference whether diabetes is the primary disease or is caused by another condition; the complications will be the same (though they are usually more severe when diabetes is the primary cause, because the blood sugar levels tend to be higher for a longer period of time).

The Patient Must Know

The more the diabetic understands his or her body and what is happening, the better the chances are of controlling the disease and preventing complications. The arm's-length distance between patient and physician must be overcome. There are more education materials and classes than ever before to help you, the patient, acquire the information you need to understand what is going on. Without a real understanding of why strict control of diet, exercise, and medication must be maintained, it is easy for you to stray from the path that you must now walk for the rest of your life.

When a patient does not follow the doctor's advice, the doctor frequently will become frustrated. However, the problem often lies with the physician who has not taken the time to explain the therapy to the patient and its importance.

For instance, since there are a number of oral agents, not all of which do the same job, the patient should know the kind specifically prescribed and what it is supposed to do.

Taking the time to do things correctly initially, including educating the patient, can be the most efficient way to bring the disease under control.

Two facts we will readily concede about the medical treatment of diabetes are that it is not easy, and that it is time-consuming. It is not easy because diabetes is a complex disease, and it is time-consuming because a medical professional must take the time to teach the diabetic about how the body normally functions as well as what is out of balance in diabetes. In addition, the diabetic needs to know how the medications work, how to check his or her own blood glucose levels, and how to adjust diet and medications when necessary.

The Diabetes Educator

For a physician with a demanding schedule, no matter how conscientious, it is a dilemma—but not an impossible one. And here's where the diabetes educator comes in. The educator is trained and knowledgeable in the day-to-day management of diabetes as well as in the principles of education.

In 1972, a group of eighteen nurses interested in specializing in this field met and formed the American Association of Diabetes Educators (AADE). It was determined that in addition to their role as nurses, they should assume teaching responsibilities. There was, they felt, a vast information gap between physicians and diabetics. Diabetics were not receiving adequate explanation and instruction as to how to keep their disease under control.

Unfortunately, there was nowhere to go to earn a degree in the field, nor was there a way for a person to become certified as a diabetes educator. That, fortunately, is no longer the case. With the help of physicians and special diabetes education courses, which are provided by diabetes research and training centers in several cities across the United States, many nurses, dietitians, and other professionals are acquiring the necessary skills to become effective diabetes educators. In addition, the AADE has developed a certification examination for professional diabetes educators.

To counsel a diabetic about diet does not require that one be a dietitian, but training in nutrition is essential. To teach diabetics new eating patterns, these educators learn to show people how to change their eating habits and to motivate them to follow their prescribed management plan. This is important for diabetics, since they have a need to learn not only *what, when,* and *how much* to eat but how the combination of diet, exercise, and medication affects their blood sugar levels.

For instance, there is a simple mealtime pattern that, if adopted, might help diabetics control their food intake. In many households the food for a meal is brought to the table in serving dishes and each person fills a plate and then begins to eat. Instead of following this pattern, the family that includes a diabetic might leave the food in the kitchen or on the stove. Then each person, especially the diabetic, puts the appropriate amount of food on his or her own plate before sitting at the table to eat. Simple yet effective in overcoming the temptation to take second and third helpings and thus overeat.

Another simple, effective method of establishing better habits involves teaching diabetics how to shop wisely for food. They can learn what *not* to bring home—behavior modification is essential.

An Understanding Ear

The educator is sometimes more sensitive than the doctor at working on the more subtle, psychological problems associated with diabetes. As the educator spends time instructing the diabetic, the educator may sense more quickly than a physician would, for instance, whether the diabetic is accepting the disease as a fact of life. As we've emphasized before, people with newly diagnosed diabetes often feel that they have lost their health and are no longer in control of their life. They may be put into a hospital, their diets are controlled, blood samples are taken, they are given insulin injections or pills, and they are faced with big words and complex concepts that they probably do not understand.

They have to cope with the fact that they can no longer eat as they please without endangering their health, and that they may, in some instances, have to take medication for the rest of their lives. This realization can be threatening and frightening.

Diabetics may at some point feel angry toward the doctor, their family, themselves, or life itself for this discouraging turn of events. There may also be a time of sadness or depression as they grieve over what might have been. They may suppress all these feelings so effectively that they may not even be aware that they are denying the reality of their situation.

Dealing with a new disease and all the feelings it creates is difficult, and the new diabetic needs a lot of support. The diabetes educator can play a very important role in helping the patient through this difficult time.

A Gradual Approach

Because this is such a difficult time, diabetics should be taught only the essentials at first. All they really want to know at this early stage is what they need to do in order to survive—what they should eat today and tomorrow and how to take their medication. Other parts of their instruction, like the importance of exercise, can come later. They simply want to know how to get through today and tomorrow.

They also need a great deal of support, and to know that the medical profession will help them learn how to care for themselves. The responsibility of the educator is (1) to identify their needs and (2) to develop a plan to teach them how to manage their diabetes on a daily basis.

As diabetics master skills that allow them to care for themselves, such as self-testing of blood glucose and meal planning, their self-esteem is restored and the power of decision-making is regained. At this point, patients usually begin to seek new learning opportunities that will provide them with more advanced information and the skills needed to increase the flexibility of their lifestyle. Actively seeking new learning opportunities is indicative of approaching successful adaptation to diabetes and signals the ending of the normal and protective grief process.

Survival Skills

The education process begins with teaching the survival skills: meal planning, self-monitoring of blood glucose, and administration of medications. How is this different from what the physician does?

Basically, the physician prescribes a treatment program, including daily caloric intake, the number of meals and snacks, the amount, type, and time of insulin injections or times to take oral agents or other medications.

The educator then teaches the patient the skills needed to *carry out* the treatment program. It is the educator (usually a nurse) who teaches the patient how to administer insulin and adjust the dosage, how to measure blood glucose levels, how to plan appropriate meals, and how to maintain good blood sugar control.

Individual attention to specific problems may help to avert misunderstandings that could lead to complications or even crises. The educator's thorough understanding of a diabetic's life patterns and needs can facilitate adjustment to, and acceptance of, the doctor's recommendations. Unlike the physician, the educator often has the time to discover if a diabetic is having more difficulty than usual in accepting and dealing with the disease; and can even recommend a specialized counselor if one is needed.

The Juvenile Diabetic

When the diabetic is a child or adolescent, extra problems may arise; here, the educator's attention and availability could be crucial. For instance, an adolescent girl with Type I diabetes may feel "her life is over" when she discovers she has the disease. She is most concerned about her peer group, how she looks, her self-image.

Perhaps she wants to be a cheerleader or participate in sports. The educator can counsel her that there is no reason why her diabetes should affect her becoming a cheerleader or athlete. Together they can plan a daily routine that will allow her to do anything she wants to do, fitting it into a planned schedule.

Peer pressure makes the girl want to fit in. Nothing, she feels, should mark her as different. The educator can help her to understand that not everyone has to know that she has diabetes. She may feel more comfortable if her best friend knows, but it certainly is not necessary to tell everyone.

She can go to the hamburger palace with her friends and, so long as she has planned for it (as we'll see in the next chapter), can enjoy many of the same things everyone else enjoys just by learning how to substitute foods.

Parents may require support and counseling more than their child does. The child may be coping just fine while the parents, not understanding that he can grow up to lead a normal independent life, react by overprotecting. The adolescent may want to go away to college, but parents are often reluctant, particularly if the child has had diabetes from an early age. They may not be able to "let go" of watching over the child's physical well-being.

In one instance, a mother telephoned an educator to report that her son was supposed to be checking his blood sugar four times a day. She went on to say that for the last 10 days she had found only two of the test strips in the trash can, but that the boy had written down four test results on his record sheet.

The educator asked where the record sheets were posted and discovered that the mother had been keeping them in plain view on the kitchen cabinet for everyone to see, check over, and comment on at dinner. The educator suggested that it was time to give the boy some privacy, to let him keep the record in his room, and that the parents and the boy come in to further discuss and develop a new self-responsibility program for the boy.

Often the educator is the best equipped psychologically to work with the parents and the child toward loosening the apron strings. He or she, usually in discussions with the patient alone, will be able to discover the true problems. As a third party, the educator can often be the best one to observe and comment on family behavior patterns that are not supportive or are even counterproductive. In addition, the glycohemoglobin test, the laboratory blood test that shows an approximate 2 to 3 month average of blood sugar levels, can be used to help the educator and physician illustrate to the patient the importance of control and consistency in diabetes management. It can also serve as an excellent benchmark of progress toward good control.

Taking Responsibility

All people, even those as young as 7 or 8, can learn to be responsible for maintaining their records, and should be actively encouraged to take responsibility for their health. It is essential that they take charge as soon as possible for the day-to-day management of their diabetes. The older they get, the less time they will spend at home. Therefore, it is important that they take that responsibility as much as possible from the start.

With children or adults the educator often starts out by doing a patient-needs assessment. He or she learns what the patient perceives as important—what the priorities are in that individual's life. That provides a lot of clues as to what approaches should be taken in this particular diabetic's education and counseling.

Listening, Counseling, Managing

It is not just children who have problems coping with diabetes. Adult diabetics, too, often have misconceptions about their disease and difficulties coping with it on a daily basis.

Let's look at the case of a thirty-five-year-old divorcee with two teenage children. She married young and may feel that the first part of her life was cut short because of that. Now she has more freedom and plans for having a good time. Then she discovers she has diabetes.

She may have met someone who is a potential husband and is faced with the problem of how to tell him she has diabetes. She may be tempted to keep it a secret. This sort of situation—where diabetes interferes with one's peace of mind—is just where the educator can step in and be of assistance. In fact, diabetics will frequently have a closer, more open relationship with the educator than with their physician. The physician is an authority figure whose time is limited. So educators will find themselves listening to patients' worries about coping, sometimes even frank confessions of sexual problems.

It is up to the educator to counsel and advise. The "boyfriend" of this 35-year-old divorcee also needs to understand why she can't eat the candy he brings her, for instance, and her other "special" situations like going out to dinner or the need to carry an insulin syringe or monitor her blood glucose. The educator will often use role-playing to help patients cope with problems that may seem monumental only to them.

Sometimes the problems are not so complicated. For example, remember the overweight truck driver who knows he will lose his job if he cannot bring his diabetes under control? In this type of situation there may not be any psychological problem that has to be overcome. It is simply a matter of motivation, motivation that he must lose weight or he may end up without a job (though knowing that, too, may be a great source of anxiety to him—anxiety he may want to get off his chest with a sympathetic professional).

It is the educator who will work out a meal plan with the diabetic, one that will not overload the pancreas. The educator can encourage and teach patients to be good self-managers. She can also teach them how to use self blood glucose monitoring. Then, together, they build the decision-making skills, learn the best times to eat as well as what to eat, and when to exercise.

The Ultimate Value of the Educator

The American Association of Diabetes Educators (AADE) is working to establish a certification process for educators. The association has developed twelve self-study courses on diabetes education. With a baseline membership of 3,000 at present in the AADE, the medical community anticipates that educator certification will result in national recognition and possibly third-party payment for this important educational service. Currently, the cost of diabetes educators' services must be incorporated into the charges for a doctor's office visit, since most insurance plans do not reimburse for education.

When this recognition is achieved, the prospect of thousands of diabetes educators assisting physicians in private practice situations will become a real possibility. With that kind of help, there could be a valuable reduction in the cost of expensive hospitalizations for educating diabetics and correcting blood sugar levels and a great improvement in management by diabetic patients.

The education of the diabetic has been shown to be cost-effective. For example, the cost of just one day in the hospital exceeds the expense of an entire year of self blood glucose monitoring.

CHAPTER 14

Normalization of Blood Glucose Levels: Diet, Exercise, and Medication

The cornerstone of treatment for all diabetics is an appropriate diet, one designed to achieve and maintain desirable body weight and to minimize elevations in blood glucose levels. To determine desirable body weight, the doctor must consider a person's sex and body build as well as height. If the patient is overweight, a weight-reducing diet has to be designed. If the patient is underweight, then he or she must go on a weight-gaining diet. Once the patient has achieved desirable body weight, then the diet is adjusted to *maintain* this ideal body mass.

There are some simple rules of thumb for estimating desirable body weight and calorie needs. As an example, a five-foot-tall female should weigh about 100 pounds. For each inch over five feet, add five pounds. Therefore, a girl who is five feet two should weigh 110 pounds. One who is five feet five should weigh 125, and so forth.

Those guidelines can be adjusted by 10 percent either way, depending on whether the person is small-framed or large-framed. For a fine-boned woman who is five feet five inches tall, the best body weight may be about 115 pounds, while for a large-framed woman of the same height, 135 may be ideal.

For a five-foot-tall man, 106 pounds is the ideal weight. For each additional inch over five feet, add six pounds. The 10 percent adjustment for difference in build applies also to men.

The physician and the patient know the target they are shooting for. Once that desirable body weight has been achieved, then it takes about 15 calories a pound per day to maintain body weight. It takes about 10 calories per pound of ideal body weight to lose weight and about 20–25 calories per pound to gain weight. Additional calories are required to meet the needs of an exercise program. Once the calorie count has been determined, then those calories are divided into three meals and three snacks a day: breakfast, mid-morning snack, lunch, mid-afternoon snack, dinner and bedtime snack.

Adapting Diet to Existing Habits

Some physicians make a mistake in handing out printed diets without regard to the food preferences and eating habits of the patient. The diet should be constructed on the basis of the diabetic's preferences (i.e., work schedule, ethnic food habits, or just whether he likes a small breakfast, small lunch and a larger evening meal or would prefer to have the calories equally distributed). Whatever the tastes, the diet must be one that the individual can live with and manage seven days a week. Once patients understand the goals and reasons, behavior modification becomes easier to accomplish.

Since a diabetic who is taking insulin needs to eat food and take insulin injections at the same time every day, seven days a week, it is best to try to adapt diet to established habits, if possible. It is also important to establish and understand the relationship of eating times to injections. Once an insulin injection is given, it cannot be removed from the system.

After injection, there is a fairly critical time period—thirty to sixty minutes—in which the diabetic must eat or run the risk of suffering insulin reaction or insulin shock when the blood sugar falls too low as the insulin processes it out of the circulatory system. Eating serves to replace that sugar as it is being "carried away" to the cells.

Once the diet has been established, then that diet plus whatever exercise program the patient and doctor have chosen will determine the times, the amounts, and the types of insulin taken. (Diet and exercise programs are equally important for all diabetics whether or not they are taking insulin.)

Adjustments

Those are the basic rules, which is not to say they cannot be adjusted. If necessary, a diabetic can manipulate diet, with the aid of an educator or dietitian. This is particularly important for someone whose activity varies from day to day. For instance, take a woman who has a part-time job. Four days a week she is at home doing housework or gardening; three days she works at a job where she sits all day. For the active days, she may be prescribed an extra 200 calories or so. That calorie adjustment would apply for any additional activity over the norm.

But, if you go on a weight-reducing diet and are consuming minimum calories, you would also take correspondingly lowered insulin doses. If you are adding more exercise as well, the insulin doses must be further adjusted. This adjustment requires careful consideration.

As discussed in Chapter 8 in relationship to morning sickness during pregnancy, one of the things that many diabetics do not realize is that their liver continues to produce glucose even if they do not eat. Diabetics may rationalize that if they do not eat, then they don't need to take insulin because their blood sugar cannot be high. It just doesn't work that way. In the absence of insulin, the liver continues to make glucose from amino acids formed from muscle breakdown. Therefore, it is important to check the urine for sugar and ketones and use self blood glucose monitoring measurements to determine the amount of insulin to take.

Determining Insulin Dosage

Once the doctor and the diabetic plan the appropriate diet, then the necessary amount of insulin must be determined. The amount of insulin prescribed initially is an educated guess. Generally an intermediate insulin (which works over an extended period of time) and regular insulin (the quick-acting type) are used in combination. The diabetic usually takes two injections a day, but the morning and evening doses are generally different. In most cases, two thirds to three fourths of the day's total dosage is taken before breakfast. After the morning injection, the diabetic follows a routine of breakfast, snack, lunch, snack—with, of course, all the day's activities between—before taking the evening dose. After that, the diabetic eats only the evening meal and a snack right before going to bed. Self blood glucose monitoring a half hour before meals helps in adjusting the insulin dose.

All too frequently, the diabetic's blood glucose is poorly controlled. In managing diabetes, the development of insulin therapy was a life saver. On the other hand, the subsequent development of long-acting insulin—the so-called one-dose-a-day insulin—was a mixed blessing, because it engendered the false impression in both physicians and patients that the disease was being well managed as long as the patient took his daily dose and avoided ketoacidosis. Today, seven out of ten individuals who have to take insulin take only one injection a day. Unfortunately, one dose does not give effective circulating blood levels of insulin for a whole day. If one takes it in the morning, the effectiveness of the injection peaks at perhaps 3:00 or 4:00 PM, or later, depending on whether it is intermediate or long-lasting insulin. By 2:00 AM, however, there is very little insulin left. Although these low levels of insulin are adequate to prevent ketoacidosis, they are insufficient to control blood sugar levels that rise, causing damage to the nerves and blood vessels.

Insulin Shock

Insulin shock is one of the greatest threats to the well being of an insulin-requiring diabetic. Back in Chapter 2, we discussed the finely-honed glucose/insulin feedback system that functions in the normal, nondiabetic person. Most diabetics realize, of course, that this system has been thwarted in their bodies. But what many do not realize is that artificially supplied insulin does not necessarily make up for all the deficiencies in that system.

In the Islets of Langerhans, you'll remember, the beta cells make insulin and the alpha cells make glucagon. These two hormones have virtually opposite effects on the body. Simply put, high blood sugar causes the pancreas to release insulin, while low blood sugar triggers the release of glucagon. (Because of this inverse function, they are known as counterregulatory hormones.)

When we eat and our blood sugar level increases, insulin is normally released by the beta cells to metabolize that sugar and maintain an even supply in the blood, promoting the uptake of glucose and amino acids by the various cells that need them. Conversely, when we fast and the blood sugar level drops, glucagon is released by the alpha cells. Glucagon promotes the rapid breakdown of the liver's glycogen to glucose which is released into the blood. Glucagon also promotes the transformation (in the liver) of amino acids (which are formed continuously by the natural breakdown of muscle) into glucose, a constant supply of which is vital to all functioning tissues, but especially to the brain.

The brain can sometimes get by on amazingly low levels of glucose without damage, but there is a limit. The limit is known as your critical hypoglycemic level. This threshold varies from one individual to another, but at that crucial point in each individual brain cells cannot function adequately to maintain consciousness. This state of severe hypoglycemia is known as insulin shock; it is, in effect, a state of coma.

In an insulin-dependent diabetic, the insulin is being supplied from outside the body's natural system. This means that if for some reason (e.g., unplanned-for rigorous exercise) the body uses up its available glucose, the natural mechanism that would cut off the supply of insulin from the beta cells in the pancreas has *no control* over the amount of insulin taken by injection.

What happens is that this injected insulin continues to be absorbed and to promote the uptake of glucose by the fat and muscle cells, leaving too little for immediate use by the brain. Even the available supply of glucagon from the alpha cells and epinephrine (from the adrenals), which also promotes conversion of amino acids into glucose by the liver, cannot compensate adequately.

What Happens to the Brain

The brain and the nerves operate mainly by a system of changing electrical potential, which is produced by differences in salt concentrations inside and outside each cell. To simplify matters, we'll say that outside the cell is sodium; inside potassium. That balance of exterior sodium to interior potassium is maintained by "pumps," which are fueled by glucose. Without adequate glucose, the "pumps" stop functioning. The sodium leaks in and mixes with the potassium inside the cell. Chaos occurs. The electrical potential is reduced and the person loses consciousness. This is insulin shock.

If this energy shortage for the "pumps" is brief, the brain can recover on its own; if it lasts too long, however, (say, several hours) permanent brain damage may result. If a person in this state is brought into an emergency room, medics will usually inject him with quick sugars or extra glucagon, to raise blood glucose levels as quickly as possible. Glucagon acts by giving the liver a boost, making it release more glucose.

Averting the Crisis

So what about the person who is alone and going into insulin shock? The answer to this question depends on the severity of the situation. If there is not too much excess insulin, then it will be broken down and metabolized, and the glucose levels will start building up again before serious damage occurs. If the brain is not deprived of glucose for too long a time, it will recover without adverse effect.

Since the effect of low sugar on brain function does vary from one individual to another and depends on the *rate* at which blood sugar drops as well as how low it drops and how long it remains low, it is virtually impossible to predict just how low the sugar has to be to have a serious effect on a given person, or at what level coma will result. Generally speaking, however, permanent brain damage is unlikely to occur in the absence of coma, or from a coma of less than 30 minutes duration. And when insulin shock does occur, doctors cannot tell until the person recovers whether the brain has been permanently damaged. (In well-managed insulin-dependent diabetics, brain damage from insulin shock is a very rare occurrence.) Obviously, insulin shock—known in its early-warning phase as insulin reaction—is a state to be avoided at all costs.

Fortunately, many people can actually sense when their blood sugar level is dropping too low. They begin to feel sweaty and nervous, and may become confused and irritable. As a result, they know they need to check their blood sugar, drink fruit juice, or take Monoject® Insulin Reaction Gel, a sugar-containing gel formulated to raise blood sugar quickly, or some other fast sugar, to avert a crisis.

However, others cannot recognize these changes and do not realize they are heading toward this dangerous state. Suddenly, they lose consciousness. When they do, they are in peril of suffering brain damage if no one is around to recognize the symptoms and to get help or administer a remedy. Members of the family and close friends must be taught to give the person an injection of glucagon or call 911 or an ambulance.

Some diabetics become combative during insulin reaction. When that happens, it may be difficult even for a knowledgeable close friend or relative to get them to cooperate by consuming a fast sugar supplement. Prevention should be the goal.

The Importance of Self-Monitoring

This brings us to the importance of routine self-monitoring of blood glucose in the prevention of hypoglycemia and insulin shock.

Self glucose monitoring is a system now widely used by many diabetics. Because of recent technological developments, the glucose monitor is becoming easier to use, is less expensive, and is a highly reliable tool for self-control and management for the diabetic.

The most important information you need to know to control your diabetes is the level of your blood sugar throughout the day. The only way to get regular, accurate information about blood sugar levels is to perform blood sugar tests. A person sticks his finger with a special lancet, obtains a drop of blood, puts the blood on a chemically treated test strip for a specified time (it varies with different systems, usually 1 minute), wipes the blood and compares the color of the test strip pad to a color chart on the back of the strip container. The chart gives color variations for blood glucose levels. Alternatively, diabetics can purchase a small, compact, calculator-size meter that has a digital display. The strips are inserted into the meter and it reads the chemical change and displays an exact blood glucose reading. Both methods are highly efficient and beneficial, however the visual (color chart) method requires adequate color vision for accurate interpretation.

Until a few years ago, diabetics could check the presence of sugar at home only be testing their urine. The telltale trace of sugar in the urine in an individual with normal renal threshold indicates that the level of sugar in the bloodstream is at least 180–200. But, as you read earlier, the renal threshold is not the same in everyone, and some people can achieve dangerously high blood sugar levels without spilling glucose into their urine at all.

In order to prevent the complications of diabetes (long-term as well as short-term), we feel that tight control of blood sugar levels is essential; they should neither rise too high nor fall too low, regardless of one's sense of immediate well-being. To accomplish such rigorous control, most diabetics cannot rely on urine tests. Some still do, with the approval of their physician, but this system is not, in our opinion, as accurate as it ought to be.* Whatever system your doctor does prescribe, however, the important thing is to use it daily and to know how to interpret the results.

Sometimes, checking the urine may be an adequate test in the beginning of treatment. Using the urine sugar results as a guide, the doctor adjusts insulin dosage accordingly. Once the doctor feels that he or she is bringing the glucose level below 200 mg/dl, blood tests can be used as a guide. If, for example, the physician knows that the patient is spilling one or

*Self monitoring of urine may, however, be perfectly adequate for youngsters who generally have thresholds lower than normal; this means that blood sugar levels just above normal may betray themselves right away in a urine sample.

two percent sugar in his urine, and his renal threshold is normal, then instead of drawing blood to test for sugars, the doctors can just increase the regular and intermediate insulins. With that done, the physician checks to see if there is a decrease in the amount of urine sugar.

If the urine sugar before the evening meal is negative, then, knowing the renal threshold, the physician can be reasonably confident that the blood sugar is probably all right, too, and that the right amount of insulin was given that same morning.

Sugar levels in the morning indicate whether the appropriate amount of insulin was taken the previous evening. To determine the exact blood sugar, however, a blood sample must be taken and measured.

Technology has improved. Self glucose monitoring devices have enabled diabetics to achieve and maintain excellent blood sugar control virtually twenty-four hours a day. Self-testing with these instruments takes only one to two minutes and gives accurate information. As a result, diabetics have reported that for the first time since they were diagnosed, they feel they have control of their lives.

Achieving Normalization without Sacrificing Variety

The aim of self-monitoring of blood sugar is to achieve normal blood sugar levels before breakfast, before lunch, and before the evening meal. Once the patient and doctor know how to normalize these levels and the patient sticks to the designated diet and physical activity program, he should be able to maintain those normal levels fairly consistently. It is not unusual for someone to maintain normal blood sugars for years without any great change, except during illnesses, infections, surgery, pregnancy, and other conditions or situations that alter metabolism. Good control requires education, self-discipline, and monitoring.

That last statement may sound a bit rigorous or confining to you. You might picture an endlessly monotonous life of schedules; boring, virtuous foods; rigorously controlled calisthenics. But for the educated diabetic, that's a far cry from reality; the more you know about the "whys" of your treatment, the more flexible you can be.

Take, for instance, that teenage girl back in Chapter 13 who is suffering from peer pressure and wants to go to a hamburger palace and eat with her friend. Can she do so without suffering any ill consequences? Yes . . . if she understands what it will take to keep her system in balance. With education and motivation, this situation poses no real dilemma to the conscientious diabetic.

It all depends very much on when and what she eats. The time must coincide with regular mealtimes or snacks. There are "exchange lists" for foods, and we'll provide you with those lists in the next chapter. The teenage girl on a diabetic diet will know just what that diet consists of; she'll know the number of bread, meat, fruit, fat, and milk exchanges she can eat. There are even charts for "fast foods".

All she has to do in this situation is take the fast food items, which are easily converted to exchanges, and substitute the items desired for corresponding foods she might have eaten at home instead. She'll have to skip the sugared soda pop and substitute a diet drink, but she is probably already doing that as an everyday habit along with many of her friends.

Inappropriate Foods

Unfortunately, despite such allowances, resistance to accepting a diabetic diet is a very common problem. Often, the typical Type II diabetic (over forty and overweight) has a passion for certain high-calorie, high-sugar foods enjoyed throughout a lifetime. In fact, he or she may very well be convinced (thanks to the myths perpetrated by those so-called experts) that if deprived of such foods, the fat cells will torture him into submission.

Individuals who have a strong desire to continue eating inappropriate foods, which are rich and sweet (i.e., candy and desserts), can put themselves through all kinds of suffering. It is essential for physicians to emphasize to such people that they have a chronic disease and that the consequences can be pretty dismal if diet—not to mention exercise and medication—are disregarded. There are some foods that just have to be avoided altogether. However, there are several cookbooks (see appendix) which offer creative alternatives which can be incorporated into the exchange lists and meal planning.

Equally problematic is a sociable person who is a diabetic and goes out once a week to bowl and have a few drinks. Bowling is not the problem for this three-hour athlete; the problem is the beer or alcohol consumption.

Alcohol and the Liver

There is nothing wrong with a diabetic having a beer or other alcoholic beverage (i.e., a glass of wine with dinner) on occasion. But three beers in one evening are too many, and a six-pack could be disastrous. First of all, one tends to forget that alcohol contains a hefty share of calories. But worse than the effect of all those calories is what the alcohol does to the liver: It decreases the liver's ability to release glucose. (This is true even for the nondiabetic.) For the diabetic whose body needs glucose because the blood sugar has dropped after an insulin injection, the effect of too much alcohol could be catastrophic. Furthermore, the person who's had one too many beers may not be alert enough to recognize an insulin reaction if there is one.

The Importance of Exercise

The Diabetic Athlete

What about flexibility in an exercise program? We just looked at the teenage girl who wants to go to a fast food restaurant; what about the teenage boy—or even grown man—who likes to play hockey in winter, soccer in spring, and baseball in summer? Does he have to give up sports if he develops diabetes? The answer, happily, is *no.*

If the diabetes is well controlled and an individual wants to engage in vigorous physical activity, he begins simply by learning the approximate calories-per-minute used up in the chosen sport. If he is going to be doing a lot of running—as in hockey, soccer or football—he will use up about 20 calories per minute. If the event takes an hour, and the individual involved figures on running for half of that time, then he will have to figure on 30 minutes times 20 calories (600 calories) expended for that time. Knowing this, he can consume an extra 600 calories before the event. Six hundred calories could be taken, for instance, in a sandwich and a glass of milk. Those calories will carry him through that hour of increased physical exertion without much risk of insulin reaction.

Calories Burned Exercising

	Calories Burned per Minute
Basketball	19
Bowling	8
Cycling	8
Golf	6
Jogging	17
Swimming	12
Tennis	7
Walking (indoors)	3
Walking (outdoors)	6
Vigorous running	20

Still, just as a precaution, he can carry packets of Monoject® Insulin Reaction Gel or other similar product to quickly raise blood sugar. If he feels an insulin reaction coming on, he can consume one of those. There have, in fact, been many instances of individuals with blood sugars in the 20s and 30s who have taken one or two of these and stopped a reaction. The person can then consume some food to bring his blood sugar up to a safe level.

One thing is certain: A diabetic cannot eat just an apple and then go out and play football, hockey, basketball, or soccer.

Even baseball, which does not require as many calories as the sports in which participants are running constantly, calls for significant additional calories.

Another aid for the diabetic athlete is a self blood glucose monitoring device (as described earlier). Within 45 seconds to two minutes of testing his blood, the diabetic can determine the blood sugar level. The individual can then adjust his or her calorie intake as appropriate.

Establishing Individual Guidelines

There are no hard and fast formulas for determining exactly how much an individual diabetic athlete should eat. You start with your best guess-timates and then work a system by trial and error. The physician provides the general guidelines, but the athlete works out the specific rules.

For instance, one guideline would be that you should guard against giving yourself an insulin injection in a muscle group that is especially exercised during your sport. For example, a tennis player would want to take his injection in his abdomen. This is just common sense. The more exercise you perform using your arms or legs, the quicker the insulin will be absorbed into the bloodstream if it is injected there. Knowing that, one can reason that the quicker the insulin enters the blood, the quicker it is going to act. So picking the wrong place for an injection before vigorous physical activity could produce an insulin reaction even with precisely the right dosage.

Before a sports event, the best place to give an injection is usually the abdomen. It is also the easiest place in which to give oneself a shot. You may have to overcome the psychological fear of sticking a needle into your belly.

The Part-Time Athlete

Ironically, the part-time athlete may have a harder time adjusting to diabetes than the regular team athlete does. Say you are a diabetic on the green side of forty and you have a son with whom you want to participate now and then in a sport. To do this, you would first have to take the same precautions as if you did not have diabetes. You would do a gradual exercise program to build up your strength and endurance, learn to do stretching exercises, and get proper equipment.

Then one element that would be different is that the part-time athlete with diabetes should try to do his sport at the same time of day every time. He should plan ahead whether he is going to run before a meal or after a meal. Jogging expends 17 calories a minute. So if you plan to run for an hour, you'll need 17 calories times 60 minutes—that's 1,020 additional calories—to meet your requirements.

Everyone with diabetes should incorporate exercise of some kind (riding a stationary bike, walking, etc.) into their daily routine.

Three Variables

The main thing to keep in mind when compensating for exercise is that it is one of three interrelated variables, the other two being diet and insulin. If you have taken insulin and *then* want to increase your physical activity, additional calories are required. By the same principles, when an overweight diabetic is on a weight-loss program including both diet and exercise, exercise can be increased while maintaining a low-calorie intake. It is very important, however, that his or her blood glucose be reasonably well controlled before undertaking a new exercise regimen.

Oral Agents: Who Is a Candidate?

Not every Type II diabetic is over forty, and not all are overweight. Often a Type II diabetic can be treated with just a diabetic diet and an exercise program. If he does not respond properly to that, then an oral agent should be prescribed. These individuals are generally patients with mild forms of Type II diabetes: Those who have blood sugar levels rarely exceeding 200. An individual with blood sugars consistently as high as 400 or 500 frequently will not respond to an oral agent.

Deciding which oral agent to use, however, is a matter of educated guessing, so physicians must closely monitor patients under consideration for this type of treatment. There is simply no reliable way to predict who will respond to which oral agent or how long a person will *continue* to respond even after initial success with a particular medication. If one oral agent does not work, another one can be tried.

A number of different agents have been developed over the years. They accomplish different things. Some promote the release of existing insulin reserves in direct response to an increase in blood glucose levels. Others increase the actual number of insulin receptors on muscle and fat cells so that the available insulin is more effective. Still others actually work on the liver, interfering with its production of glucose and thereby keeping down levels of sugar in the bloodstream. They are not an oral form of insulin.

Although most diabetics do respond well to insulin injections *or* to oral agents, some may benefit from a combination. These individuals are often grossly overweight. Instead of giving them larger and larger doses of insulin, their doctors may prescribe a low insulin dose combined with an oral agent. If they lose weight, they are taken off the insulin and may be maintained on oral agents exclusively. If they continue to lose weight, they may reach a point when they do not need even the oral agents and their pancreas once again functions adequately to metabolize sugars and maintain normal glucose levels.

Monitoring the Effectiveness of Medication

The best way to check on the effectiveness of a particular oral agent is for the diabetic to keep in contact with the doctor and educator and to keep an eye on his progress between visits by checking his urine for sugar four times a day or, as we recommend, using one of the newer self blood glucose monitoring systems to check the sugar before each meal and at bedtime. Usually improvement is seen within a week after starting treatment.

If, for instance, the urine sugar diminishes but still is not negative or the blood sugar levels are not below 150 mg/dl after a few weeks, the individual's doctor will probably want to increase the dose or switch to a different type of medication.

Some individuals have been able to control their diabetes with oral agents for decades. But any oral agent may lose its effectiveness, and that is why diabetics must be periodically monitored by medically trained professionals. If a diabetic does become unresponsive to an oral agent, his or her doctor may want to switch to another agent before resorting to insulin. Other individuals respond to an oral agent by developing hypoglycemia. A good physician never writes a prescription for an oral agent and then says to the patient, "See you in six months."

Ultimately, if an individual does not respond to oral agents, he or she must be switched to an appropriate combination of diet, exercise, and insulin, in which case the principles of treatment would be the same as for a Type I diabetic.

Are Oral Agents Dangerous?

Some doctors have expressed fears that oral agents are potentially dangerous. Well, that is true; but then, it is also true for just about any other medication you can think of—heart medicines and antibiotics, for instance. However, the key word here is *potentially.* Practically speaking, oral agents are not dangerous at all if used as directed under the supervision of a competent physician.

Breaking the Routine

The importance of adhering to a routine schedule for meals, exercise, and medication has been stressed, but perhaps not strongly enough. Once a diabetic establishes regular schedules, he is less likely to have an insulin reaction or to get out of control.

But even the most conscientious person can be faced with an unexpected break in routine. For instance, it is sometimes necessary for a person to leave home for a week or two, during which time it may very well, by unavoidable circumstances, be impossible to maintain the regular eating and exercise schedule followed at home.

Still, the individual can adjust for that kind of break in normal activity. That is one of the advantages of taking two or more insulin shots a day, rather than just one, and of using self monitoring of blood sugar. A person can always change the times and adjust the dosage of the second shot to compensate for unanticipated changes in the time of the evening meal or in physical activity, IF he knows what his blood sugar is and ONLY AFTER he has been educated in how to make these adjustments. Of course, the morning shot could be adjusted as well. If, for instance, a person was aware in advance that he would be increasing his physical activity, he could choose not to take in more calories, but inject less insulin.

What makes it so hard to convince some people of the importance of adhering to the diet-and-exercise program and taking medications is the fact that their disease is virtually pain-free for many years until complications develop.

Doctors encounter the same difficulties here that they do when trying to convince an unwilling cigarette smoker to stop smoking. Somehow those late complications are so far down the road that they seem not to have enough reality for the person intent on momentary pleasures. This is why, again, education is so essential for the diabetic who will quickly learn that the routines he can so easily learn to follow will interfere far less with enjoying life than will the consequences of neglecting them.

CHAPTER 15

Planning the Diet

One of the most important keys to successful management of diabetes is meal planning, and one of the most useful aids in planning a healthy diet is the exchange list. These lists—of which there are six—include almost every type of food, and once you understand the principle of how they work, the mental mountain that the word *diet* conjures up is brought down to eye level.*

When some people hear the word *exchange,* they imagine that this means they will be able to exchange foods they dislike for foods they like. Unfortunately, however, that is generally not the case. On the other hand, there is no reason why a diabetic should have to eat foods that are disliked. It would be more accurate to think of these lists as offering a large variety of foods with comparable nutritional value that most of us eat every day. You are free to "exchange" any food with a preferred

*We have not attempted to list all the foods that could comprise a given list, rather to provide a sample of the types of foods included. Consult the Appendix for a list of cookbooks and other sources which can provide a more varied list of exchanges and meal plans. Our thanks to Cathy Feldmeier, R.D. for her assistance.

food in that same category to constitute your requirements for each meal and snack.

Each of the six exchange lists represents a different nutritional category of food, as follows:

Bread	Breads, cereals and starchy vegetables
Meat	Lean meats, medium-fat meats, high-fat meats, and cheeses, eggs, dried beans, and peanut butter
Fat	Monounsaturated, polyunsaturated, and saturated (butter, salad dressings, bacon, oils, etc.)
Milk	Non-fat, low-fat, whole milk, and yogurt
Fruit	Fruits, fruit juices
Vegetables	Non-starchy vegetables

Each list shows equivalent amounts of foods of similar composition and caloric content within a given category. For instance, on the fruit list a third cup of prune juice is equal to 12 large cherries, which is equal to 2 medium plums, which is equal to 2 small tangerines and so on. If you don't like prune juice (some people do), there is an infinite variety of other fruits with equal carbohydrate and caloric value from which to choose.

Following the lists are some instructions for incorporating them into your meal planning. Remember, seasonings can be used with no limits (sodium is the exception) and can greatly improve the taste of foods.

Bread and Starch Exchanges

Each exchange item listed has 15 grams of carbohydrates, 3 grams of protein, and 80 calories. In general, each is one serving. *Note:* whole grain breads and starchy vegetables are good sources of fiber.

Breads:

White	1 slice
Whole wheat	1 slice

Rye	1 slice
Pumpernickel	1 slice
Raisin	1 slice
Bagel, small	1/2
English muffin	1/2
Plain roll	1
Hot dog/hamburger bun	1/2
Dried bread crumbs	3 Tbsp.
Tortilla, 6 inch	1

Cereals:

Bran flakes	1/2 cup
Other unsweetened cereals	3/4 cup
Puffed wheat and rice	1 1/2 cup
Wheat germ	3 Tbsp.
Oatmeal, cream of wheat, grits (cooked)	1/2 cup
Rice (cooked)	1/3 cup
Cornmeal (dry)	2 1/2 Tbsp.
Flour	2 1/2 Tbsp.
Popcorn (popped, no fat)	3 cups

Pastas:

Spaghetti, noodles, macaroni, (cooked)	1/2 cup

Crackers:

Graham (2 1/2-inch square)	3
Matzoth (4 by 6 inches)	1/2
Oyster	24
Rye	3
Saltines	6
Soda (2 1/2-inch square)	4
Pretzels (small sticks)	25
Vanilla wafers	6

Starchy Vegetables:

Dried beans (cooked)	1/3 cup
Dried peas (cooked)	1/3 cup
Dried lentils (cooked)	1/3 cup
Baked beans (canned vegetarian)	1/4 cup
Corn	1/2 cup
Corn on the cob (small)	1
Green peas (fresh, canned, frozen)	1/2 cup
Lima beans	1/2 cup
Parsnips	1 cup
Potato (small white)	1
Potato (mashed)	1/2 cup
Pumpkin	1 cup
Squash (winter, acorn, butternut)	3/4 cup
Yam or sweet potato	1/3 cup

Prepared Foods:

When selecting from the following Bread sublist, the figure in parentheses indicates the extra fat exchanges present in the serving that also must be counted in tabulating the total calories consumed. Thus, for example, since one fat exchange is equivalent to 45 calories, one biscuit contributes 125 calories toward the diet, not just the 80 calories in one bread exchange.

Biscuit (1), 2-inch diameter	1
Cornbread (1) 2x2x1-inch piece	1
Crackers (1) round butter type	5
Muffin (1) plain small	1
Potatoes (1) 3 1/2-inch french fries	8
Potato chips (2)	15
Corn chips (2)	15
Pancake (1) 5 1/2-inch	1
Waffle (1) 5 1/2-inch	1

From the Bread list, the following are good sources of:

Iron and Thiamin:

Whole grain and enriched breads, cereals, wheat germ, bran, dried beans, dried peas.

Fiber:

Whole grain breads, bran cereals, wheat germ, dried beans and peas, corn.

Potassium:

Wheat germ, bran, dried beans, potatoes, lima beans, parsnips, pumpkin, winter squash.

Meat Exchanges

Note: Some high-protein non-meat foods (e.g., cheeses, eggs, peanut butter) are *included* here because they will provide the same nutritional benefits as meat and can therefore be used as substitutes in this category.

All meat should be boiled, baked, broiled or barbequed. Use nonstick pan or pan spray. Trim off fat *before* cooking. Do not add breading or coating. Weigh meats *after* cooking.

Lean Meats:

One exchange of lean meat (1 Ounce) contains 7 grams of protein, 3 grams of fat and 55 calories.

Beef:

Chipped beef	1 Ounce
Tenderloin, round, sirloin	1 Ounce
Flank steak	1 Ounce

Pork:

Ham	1 Ounce
Tenderloin	1 Ounce
Canadian bacon	1 Ounce

Veal:

Chops	1 Ounce
Roast	1 Ounce
Shoulder	1 Ounce

Poultry/Game: (Without skin, low in saturated fat and cholesterol)

Chicken	1 Ounce
Cornish Hen	1 Ounce
Turkey	1 Ounce
Duck, goose, rabbit, squirrel, pheasant, venison	1 Ounce

Fish: (Low in saturated fat and cholesterol)

Any fresh or frozen fish (not breaded)	1 Ounce
Tuna (canned in water)	1/4 cup
Crab, lobster, shrimp, clams, scallops	2 Ounces
Oysters	6
Sardines	2

Miscellaneous:

Cheese—diet	1 Ounce
Cottage cheese	1/4 cup
Grated parmesan	2 Tbsp.

Medium-Fat Meats:

One exchange of Medium-Fat meat (1 Ounce) contains 7 grams of protein, 5 grams of fat and 75 calories.

Beef:

Ground	1 Ounce
Chuck, rump roast	1 Ounce
Steaks—Porterhouse, T-bone	1 Ounce

Pork:

Cutlets	1 Ounce
Loin	1 Ounce
Shoulder	1 Ounce

Lamb:

Chops, leg, roast	1 Ounce

Veal:

Cutlets	1 Ounce

Poultry:

Chicken (with skin)	1 Ounce

Fish:

Tuna, salmon (in oil, drained)	1/4 cup

Miscellaneous:

Ricotta cheese	1/4 cup
Mozzarella, Farmer's, Neufchatel cheese	1 Ounce
Egg (high in cholesterol)	1
Liver, kidney, heart, sweetbreads	1 Ounce

High-Fat Meats:

One exchange of High-Fat meats (1 Ounce) contains 7 grams of protein, 8 grams of fat and 100 calories.

Beef:

Brisket	1 Ounce
Corned Beef	1 Ounce
Rib roast	1 Ounce
Club, rib steaks	1 Ounce

Pork:

Spare ribs	1 Ounce
Pork-ground or sausage	1 Ounce

Lamb:

Patties	1 Ounce

Fish:

Any fried fish	1 Ounce

Miscellaneous:

Cheese—cheddar, swiss, blue, American	1 Ounce
Cold cuts	1 Ounce
Knockwurst, bratwurst	1 Ounce
Hot dog (chicken or turkey)	1
Hot dog (beef or pork—add one fat exchange)	1
Peanut butter	1 Tbsp.

From the Meat list, all meats are good sources of protein, and many are good sources of Iron, Zinc, Vitamin B-12, and other vitamins of the B-complex.

Oysters are high in Zinc. There is Zinc, too, in crab, liver, lean meats, and the dark meat of the turkey.

Fat Exchanges

One fat exchange contains 5 grams of fat and 45 calories.

Polyunsaturated or Monounsaturated fats:

Avocado	1/8 medium
Mayonnaise	1 tsp.
Margarine	1 tsp.
Oil (corn, cottonseed, safflower, soy, sunflower)	1 tsp.
Olives	5 large
Nuts (peanuts)	10 large, 20 small
Pecans, Walnuts (shelled)	2 whole
Salad dressings (creamy)	2 tsp.
Salad dressings (French or Italian type)	1 Tbsp.
Salad dressings (reduced calorie)	2 Tbsp.

Saturated Fats:

Butter	1 tsp.
Bacon fat	1 tsp.

Bacon	1 strip
Cream (light)	2 Tbsp.
Cream (heavy)	1 Tbsp.
Coffee creamer, powdered	4 tsp.
Cream cheese	1 Tbsp.
Sour cream	2 Tbsp.

Milk Exchanges

One exchange of milk contains 12 grams of carbohydrate, 8 grams of protein, and fat and calories as indicated.

Skim and low-fat milk: (a trace of fat and 90 calories)

Skim, 1/2%, 1% milk	1 cup
Powdered, non-fat	1/3 cup
Evaporated skim milk	1/2 cup
Buttermilk, low-fat	1 cup
Yogurt (from skim milk, plain)	1 cup

Low-fat fortified milk: (5 grams of fat, 120 calories)

2% milk	1 cup
Yogurt (from 2% milk, plain)	1 cup

Whole milk: (8 grams of fat, 150 calories)

Whole milk	1 cup
Evaporated milk	1/2 cup
Buttermilk	1 cup
Yogurt (from whole milk, plain)	1 cup

Milk is the leading source of Calcium, and is a good source of phosphorus, protein, some B-complex vitamins, Vitamin A and D and Magnesium.

Fruit Exchanges

One exchange of fruit contains 15 grams of carbohydrate and 60 calories. Choose raw or fruit packed in natural juice or water.

Apple (small)	1
Apple Juice	1/2 cup
Applesauce (unsweetened)	1/2 cup
Apricots, fresh (medium)	4
Apricots (dried)	4 halves
Banana	1/2
Berries	3/4 cup
Strawberries	1 1/4 cup
Cantaloupe (small)	1/3 melon
Cherries (large)	12
Cider	1/2 cup
Dates	2 1/2
Figs (dried)	1 1/2 cup
Grapefruit	1/2
Grapefruit Juice	1/2 cup
Grapes (any type)	15
Grape Juice	1/3 cup
Honeydew (medium)	1/8
Mango (small)	1/2
Nectarine (small)	1
Orange (small)	1
Orange Juice	1/2 cup
Papaya	1 cup
Peach (medium)	1
Pear (medium)	1
Pineapple (canned)	1/3 cup
Pineapple (raw)	3/4 cup
Pineapple juice	1/2 cup

Plum (medium)	2
Prunes (medium)	3
Prune Juice	1/3 cup
Raisins	2 Tbsp.
Tangerines (small)	2
Watermelon	1 1/4 cup

Vitamin C (good source):

Citrus fruits, raspberries, strawberries, mangoes, cantaloupes, honeydews, and papayas.

Vitamin A:

Fresh or dried apricots, mangoes, cantaloupes, nectarines, peaches.

Potassium:

Apricots, bananas, berries, grapefruit, mangoes, peaches, cantaloupes, honeydews, nectarines and oranges.

Vegetable Exchanges

One vegetable exchange has 5 grams of carbohydrate, 2 grams of protein and approximately 25 calories.

Asparagus	1/2 cup cooked (1 cup raw)
Bean Sprouts	1/2 cup cooked (1 cup raw)
Beets	1/2 cup cooked (1 cup raw)
Broccoli	1/2 cup cooked (1 cup raw)
Brussels sprouts	1/2 cup cooked (1 cup raw)
Cabbage	1/2 cup cooked (1 cup raw)
Cauliflower	1/2 cup cooked (1 cup raw)
Celery	1/2 cup cooked (1 cup raw)
Eggplant	1/2 cup cooked (1 cup raw)
Green pepper	1/2 cup cooked (1 cup raw)
Greens (all types)	1/2 cup cooked (1 cup raw)
Mushrooms	1/2 cup cooked (1 cup raw)
Okra	1/2 cup cooked (1 cup raw)

Onions	1/2 cup cooked (1 cup raw)
Rhubarb	1/2 cup cooked (1 cup raw)
Sauerkraut	1/2 cup cooked (1 cup raw)
String beans	1/2 cup cooked (1 cup raw)
Summer squash	1/2 cup cooked (1 cup raw)
Tomatoes	1/2 cup cooked (1 cup raw)
Tomato juice	1/2 cup
Turnips	1/2 cup cooked (1 cup raw)
Vegetable juice cocktail	1/2 cup
Zucchini	1/2 cup cooked (1 cup raw)

The following raw vegetables can be eaten as desired within reason without using up any exchanges:

Chinese cabbage
Cucumber
Endive
Escarole
Parsley
Dill pickles
Radishes
Spinach
Watercress

Vitamin C (good source):

Asparagus, broccoli, brussels sprouts, cabbage, cauliflower, kale, greens, spinach, tomatoes, and turnips.

Vitamin A:

Dark green and deep yellow vegetables.

Potassium:

Broccoli, brussels sprouts, beet greens, and tomato juice.

Vitamin B-6:

Broccoli, brussels sprouts, cauliflower, spinach, sauerkraut, tomatoes

Fiber is found in all vegetables.

Knowing the Numbers

These lists may remind you of the first day in algebra class; remember when you looked at the blackboard and saw: A + B = C? It did not make sense until A and B were given numerical values. Once you knew that A equaled 2 and B equaled 3, then it did not take much skill to calculate that C was 5.

That's the way the exchange lists work. Carbohydrates, Proteins, and Fats are the three major energy sources in food. The number of calories in any food item expresses its energy value. Suppose for instance, that your physician or educator presents you with an 1,800-calorie-a-day meal plan. Since we want to reduce the strain on the pancreas, we divide those 1,800 calories into three meals and three snacks. The calories should be distributed into about a 50 percent Carbohydrate, 20 percent Protein, 30 percent Fat ratio. When possible, exchanges should be lower in cholesterol and saturated fats. Cholesterol has been shown to be a risk for heart and blood vessel disease. See pages 164–167.

Your meal plan calls for:

Breakfast:
2 Bread Exchanges
1 Meat Exchange
1 Milk Exchange
1 Fruit Exchange
1 Fat Exchange

Lunch:
2 Bread Exchanges
2 Meat Exchanges
1 Fat Exchange
1 Fruit Exchange

Supper:
2 Bread Exchanges
4 Meat Exchanges
2 Vegetable Exchanges
1 Fruit Exchange
2 Fat Exchanges

AM Snack:
1 Bread Exchange
1/2 Meat

Afternoon Snack:
1/2 bread
1/2 milk

Bedtime Snack:
1 Bread Exchange
1 Meat Exchange
1 Fruit Exchange

The 430 calorie breakfast:

Calories			
160	2 bread exchanges	=	3/4 cup unsweetened cereal
			1 slice whole wheat toast
90	1 milk exchange	=	8 oz. skim milk
75	1 meat exchange	=	1 soft boiled egg
60	1 fruit exchange	=	3/4 cup blackberries
45	1 fat exchange	=	1 tsp. margarine

The 120 calorie morning snack:

80	1 bread exchange	=	1/2 bagel
40	1/2 meat exchange	=	1/2 oz. cheese

The 415 calorie lunch:

160	2 bread exchanges	=	2 slices whole wheat bread
150	2 meat exchanges	=	2 oz. ham
45	1 fat exchange	=	1 Tbsp. Italian salad dressing
60	1 fruit exchange	=	1 peach
0	coffee, tea or diet soda		
0	lettuce, pickles, and mustard for sandwich		
0	lettuce and cucumber for salad		

The 85 calorie afternoon snack:

40	1/2 bread exchange	=	3 vanilla wafers
45	1/2 milk exchange	=	1/2 cup skim milk

The 580 calorie dinner:

Calories		
160	2 bread exchanges	= 1 small baked potato
		1 small roll
220	4 lean-meat exchanges	= 4 oz. baked chicken breast
50	2 vegetable exchanges	= 1 cup broccoli
60	1 fruit exchange	= 1 1/4 cup strawberries
90	2 fat exchanges	= 1 tsp. margarine
		2 Tbsp. sour cream

The 195 calorie bedtime snack:

80	1 bread exchange	= 10 wheat thin crackers
55	1 meat exchange	= 1 oz. low-fat cheese
60	1 fruit exchange	= 15 grapes

Total 1825 calories for the day. A few over, but still within the 1800-calorie-a-day guidelines.

Cholesterol and Saturated Fat Content of Various Foods

	Portion Size	Cholesterol (mg)	Saturated Fat (g)	Saturated Fat Calories
Fats and oils				
Butter	1 tbsp	31	7	63
Lard	1 tbsp	12	5	45
Shortening				
Animal and vegetable	1 tbsp	7	5	45
Vegetable	1 tbsp	0	3	27
Tallow (beef fat), edible	1 tbsp	14	6	54
Margarine				
Corn oil (stick)	1 tbsp	0	2	18
Soybean	1 tbsp	0	2	18
Corn oil (tub)	1 tbsp	0	2	18
Soybean oil (tub)	1 tbsp	0	2	18
Margarine, diet	1 tbsp	0	1	9

	Portion Size	Cholesterol (mg)	Saturated Fat (g)	Saturated Fat Calories
Oils				
Coconut	1 tbsp	0	12	108
Corn	1 tbsp	0	2	18
Olive	1 tbsp	0	2	18
Palm	1 tbsp	0	7	63
Palm kernel	1 tbsp	0	11	99
Peanut	1 tbsp	0	2	18
Safflower	1 tbsp	0	1	9
Soybean (partially hydrogenated)	1 tbsp	0	2	18
Sunflower	1 tbsp	0	1	9
Related products				
Mayonnaise	1 tbsp	8	2	18
Peanut butter	1 tbsp	0	2	18
Dairy products				
American cheese	1 oz	27	6	54
Cheddar cheese	1 oz.	30	6	54
Cottage cheese				
Creamed, 4% fat	1 cup	34	6	54
Low-fat, 1% fat	1 cup	10	2	18
Cream	1 oz	31	6	54
Mozzarella (made with part skim)	1 oz	16	3	27
Parmesan, grated	1 tbsp	4	1	9
Swiss	1 oz	26	5	45
Cream—Half and Half™	1 tbsp	10	2	18
Cream, sour	1 tbsp	5	2	18
Cream products				
Imitation (contains coconut or palm kernel)	1/2 fl oz	0	1	9
Milk				
Whole, 3.3% fat	1 cup	33	5	45
Low-fat, 2% fat	1 cup	18	3	27
Low-fat, 1% fat	1 cup	10	2	18
Nonfat skim	1 cup	5	0.4	4
Buttermilk, cultured	1 cup	9	1	9
Milk dessert, frozen				
Regular ice cream, 10% fat	1 cup	59	9	81
Ice milk				
Soft serve, 2.6% fat	1 cup	13	3	27
Sherbert, 2% fat	1 cup	14	2	18

Cholesterol and Saturated Fat Content of Various Foods (cont'd)

	Portion Size	Cholesterol (mg)	Saturated Fat (g)	Saturated Fat Calories
Yogurt				
Made with low-fat milk	1 cup	11	2	18
Fish, shellfish, meat, and poultry (cooked)				
Beef				
Chuck arm pot roast, cooked lean	3 oz	85	3	27
Chuck blade, lean	3 oz	90	5	45
Flank, lean	3 oz	60	5	45
Rib (6–12)	3 oz	69	5	45
Rib eye (10–12)	3 oz	68	4	36
Rib (6–9)	3 oz	70	5	45
Round, full	3 oz	70	2	18
Round, bottom	3 oz	81	3	27
Round, eye	3 oz	59	2	18
Round tip, lean	3 oz	69	2	18
Round top, lean	3 oz	72	2	18
Tenderloin, lean	3 oz	72	3	27
Top loin	3 oz	65	3	27
Sirloin	3 oz	76	3	27
Ground beef, 15% fat	3 oz	70	5	45
Ground beef, 20% fat	3 oz	74	7	63
Pork				
Center rib roast chop				
Lean and fat	3 oz	69	7	63
Lean only	3 oz	67	4	36
Sirloin roast	3 oz	83	4	36
Canadian bacon	2 slices	27	1	9
Spareribs, lean and fat	2 slices	103	10	90
Cured bacon	3 slices	16	3	27
Veal cutlets	3 oz	86	4	36
Lamb loin chop, lean only	3 oz	80	4	36
Poultry				
Dark meat without skin	3 oz	79	2	18
Light meat without skin	3 oz	72	1	9

	Portion Size	Cholesterol (mg)	Saturated Fat (g)	Saturated Fat Calories
Fish				
Flounder or sole, lean fish	3 oz	59	0.3	3
Salmon, red fatty fish	3 oz	60	1	9
Shellfish				
Shrimp	3 oz	134	0.2	2
Lobster, northern	3 oz	90	0.1	1
Oyster	3 oz	45	0.5	5
Related products				
Frankfurter, beef	1	27	7	63
Bologna, beef	1 slice	16	3	27
Salami	1 slice	18	2	18
Braunschweiger	1 slice	44	3	27
Egg yolk, large	1	274	2	18
Egg white, large	1	Trace	0	0
Baked goods				
Cake, frosted				
Devil's food, frosted	1/12 8″ layer	50	5	45
Yellow cake, frosted	1/12 8″ layer	36	3	27
Brownie with icing	1	13	2	18
Chocolate chip cookies	4 cookies	21	4	27
Doughnuts, cake	1	10	1	9
Doughnuts, yeast	1	13	3	27

Free Foods

Any food or beverage that contains less than 20 calories is considered a "free food" for an exchange plan.

Coffee, tea, sugar-free soft drinks, bouillon, sugar-free drink mixes

Cabbage, celery, cucumber, green onion, mushrooms, radishes, salad greens (endive, escarole, iceberg and romaine lettuce, spinach), zucchini

Sugar-free gelatin, gum, candy, jams or jellies, syrup, and sugar substitutes

Condiments such as catsup (1 Tbsp.), mustard, horseradish, pickles (unsweetened), low-calorie salad dressings (2 Tbsp.), vinegar, taco sauce (1 Tbsp.)

CHAPTER 16

Alleviating Stress

You are swimming in the surf in the ocean. The sun is high, the sky is clear, and you are having a good time. Suddenly, you think you see the fin of a shark breaking the surface of the water. Momentarily you are paralyzed by fear. Then you react and swim for shore faster than you ever thought you could. Once on land you stand breathing hard, looking out toward the water to see if it was a shark or just your imagination that brought you back to the beach so rapidly.

Your body has reacted to fear, to stress.

You have been at the same job for 10 years, working hard for a promotion. Instead of being selected to head the department, someone from the outside is brought in and put over you. To the initial anger is added resentment and you feel terrible.

Your body is reacting to this anger, to stress.

Adrenaline Goes to Work

What is occurring within the body under stress—whether it is a single dramatic event or a nagging emotional problem—is that the adrenal glands and the nerve endings are secreting a stress hormone called epinephrine, more commonly known as adrenaline. It gives our body a boost to make it move quickly when we are startled or feel threatened.

Technically, adrenaline acts upon the tone of the muscles and on the liver, increasing glucose release. In the fat tissue it accelerates the breakdown of fats. In other words, your body is mobilizing fuel for energy to respond to a threatening situation.

If the situation is an acute, short-lived one, health consequences are usually unimportant. They may be beneficial, in fact, especially if your body's reaction had helped to save your life or prevent a serious injury.

Adrenal Corticosteroids and the Diabetic

However, if you are under continuing or recurring emotional stress, then your adrenal glands are releasing not only epinephrine but adrenal corticosteroids as well. The corticosteroids interfere with glucose metabolism by decreasing the sensitivity of tissues to insulin.

In the nondiabetic, the body can compensate for this effect. However, the diabetic can face serious problems when the tissues become resistant to insulin. These anti-insulin effects throw metabolism out of balance, and blood glucose levels go up.

In a noninsulin-dependent diabetic, severe stress can sometimes throw control off to such an extent that the individual is forced to take insulin until the situation improves.

If you are bouncing back and forth between stress and nonstress, it becomes very difficult to adjust your insulin dosage and food intake to maintain normal blood sugar levels. However, using self blood glucose monitoring can help you know what effect stress has on your blood sugar. If the insulin dose and food intake are planned for the relaxed state, then, when serious stress occurs, your body becomes less sensitive to insulin, and blood sugars may go up dramatically. You'll then need more insulin.

If you adjust your insulin dosage to compensate and then the source of stress disappears, it follows that your insulin will be out of adjustment again, perhaps causing dangerously *low* glucose levels.

Diabetics with *chronic* personal, marital, family, or job-related problems often have a very difficult time normalizing their blood sugars. They are faced with consistently fluctuating stress situations in which anti-insulin effects are constantly changing. The reason they usually cannot maintain normal glucose levels is fairly obvious. They are almost never in a stable state of metabolism.

Controlling Stress

Each of us *can* reduce the stress in our life. Stress is not an external factor. Stress exists inside us and therefore is generally subject to our control. Even when stress hits, as it often does, in response to an external event, we can usually do something. Even if we cannot change our environment, we have the option of changing the way we respond to it.

There are many ways to alter our responses to stress-provoking events. But first we must learn to recognize both the physical and the mental signs of stress (e.g., tightness in the neck or shoulder muscles, clenched jaw, a harried feeling, anger, obsession with an unpleasant event). Then we must try to identify the event(s) that brought about that response. How we perceive that event greatly determines how we respond to it.

Our perception of the meaning of events is based on what we believe—about how dependent we are on other persons, how perfect we or others should be, whether or not we have the right to get angry, what things we or others should or should not do. If our thinking and perceptions of other people and events are inaccurate or distorted, we may be causing ourselves a lot of unnecessary anguish and stress. Clarification of our beliefs can reduce the stress we feel.

For instance, do you believe you have the right to get angry? Many people have been brought up in families in which they were never allowed to express their feelings or their anger. What they do is hold all this anger inside until they finally explode. Consequently, they seethe all the time—like the person we talked about at the beginning of the chapter who lost out on a promotion to an outsider.

It is important to recognize the cause of your stress. When unexpressed feelings or anger are the cause, you must tell yourself (and believe it) that there is nothing wrong with having those feelings and expressing them appropriately. Realize, too, that you can express those feelings of anger *without feeling guilty.* Guilt may, after all, create still another source of unnecessary stress.

That kind of approach—recognition of stress and a civilized expression of anger—can benefit most people tremendously. They learn not to feel guilty about having feelings, and they learn how to express those feelings without attacking somebody. They learn to say in a straight-forward way, "I felt hurt when you said that," or "I felt intimidated when you did that." This honest, straight-forward expression of feelings can be equally helpful to the person who usually swallows all his feelings without expression (only to seethe inside) as well as to the person whose typical response is a fiery outburst that hurts and denigrates other people.

Other Ways of Coping

Such methods of controlling stressful responses can be very important to a person who has to deal with a troublesome co-worker or supervisor or who has a chronic problem at home. Learning to cope with stress may prevent headaches, high blood pressure, or ulcers that can develop.

A diabetic who learns to cope with stress by respecting and expressing feelings may also prevent wide fluctuations in blood sugar levels. Following are other ways in which one might subdue a stressful response to one's environment:

1. Exercise helps to control blood glucose levels. Moreover, it is itself an excellent way of reducing stress. When people are exercising, their mind is most often concentrated on their bodies and not on the troublesome situations with which they must cope. When the mind is applied to physical work—like running, tennis, swimming, or bicycling—the world becomes less complex, less stressful.
2. Learning to relax: Using reciprocal contraction and relaxation of muscles helps to recognize the feelings of tenseness. For example, lie flat on your back and tell first the toes, then the legs, and then the arms, neck, and face to relax. With practice, this can help you recognize that you have control over your body and your body's responses to stress.
3. Another way to relax is to develop a sense of concentration. For instance, concentrate on an eye by looking into the mirror at the pupil, and tell yourself to become calm.
4. Imaging: Concentrate on calm mental pictures in which there is no place for stress.
5. Focus on the good things. We are not suggesting that anyone strike the attitude of a Pollyanna, mostly because it would not work. However, if we allow our minds to focus on the positive side of situations, the negative aspects often diminish. Moreover, the concentration will take the focus off the problems, and help to remove the stress.

Other ways of lowering stress include yoga, biofeedback, and meditation. In general, learn to be kind to yourself by relaxing and avoiding a perfectionist's stance in which the demands you place on yourself are greater than anyone else's expectations. Respect and take care of yourself; you are the only one you will have for your entire life.

Learn to change stressful aspects of the environment that can be changed, and accept those things that cannot be changed. In short, stop beating your head against a wall.

CHAPTER 17

The Newest Approaches

We live in a period of rapidly advancing technology, a lot of which is directly and indirectly aiding medicine. Consequently, the more we learn, the more hope there is for the future, and that is certainly true in the field of diabetes.

These advances in care and treatment are most welcome. But, the notion that miraculous cures and treatments for diabetes are going to be available tomorrow can be dangerous. As we have stated before, diabetes is a very complex disease linked to hereditary and environmental factors. Diabetics, for instance, can become so certain that a "cure" for their disease is just around the corner that they may not take advantage of treatment methods already available. They rationalize that it would be much easier to achieve good control of their blood sugars with the new techniques being promised, so they wait passively. Or, they "jump" at every new idea, whether proved or not, before consulting their physician for the best advice for them.

If the technology and knowledge *currently* available are taken advantage of, they will provide most diabetics with a near normal life expectancy with minimal complications. It is foolhardy not to take advantage of available treatment while waiting or hoping for something that does not yet exist.

Later in this chapter, we will discuss the progress being made in transplant surgery and in development of new medications. But before we do, we want to emphasize the great advances made in developing new tools for management of insulin-dependent diabetes.

New Technology

The New Needles

When clinicians developed the original one-shot-a-day treatment, using long-lasting insulins, part of the rationale was to minimize the discomfort of multiple daily injections; in those days, the needles were quite painful.

In the last several years, however, the needles themselves have been improved considerably. They are now smaller and much sharper, and therefore cause minimal discomfort. In addition, they are cheaper and made to be disposable (minimizing chances of infection). Hence, taking multiple insulin injections should no longer be a source of dread for anyone.

Insulin Pumps

In the past few years, we have also seen the introduction of insulin pumps. There are external and internal varieties, although very few internal pumps are currently in use. As the popularity of pumps has grown, their cost has decreased. In addition, they have been miniaturized and are easier to wear than they once were.

The purpose of the insulin pump is to mimic the action of the pancreas by continuously secreting insulin mechanically on demand to maintain blood glucose levels within a normal range twenty-four hours a day. The two modes of operation of the pump are referred to as *Basal* and *Bolus.* The Basal infusion provides continuous delivery of small amounts of insulin to control blood glucose between meals. The Bolus infusion is the additional burst of insulin needed at mealtimes, or when blood glucose rises due to other factors.

Pumps come with an important warning: They are not a cure and they are not appropriate for all diabetics. Even patients who can use them must continue to maintain diet and exercise programs prescribed by the physician, and to check their blood glucose levels frequently so that appropriate adjustments in the insulin dosage can be made.

The External Pump

The external pump is a mechanical/electronic device (some about the size of a pack of cigarettes) worn close to the body at the waist twenty-four hours a day. It delivers the insulin from a reservoir (a syringe inside the pump) into the body by means of a flexible plastic tube connected to a needle inserted under the skin of the abdomen.

It is not entirely clear yet if external pumps offer a significant advantage over multiple injections. More and more physicians are apparently recognizing that if they were to spend as much time teaching a patient how to make the best use of multiple injections as they do on instruction about the use of a pump, the benefits would be the same. In addition, the diabetic who does not use the external pump has the advantage of not having a needle constantly under the skin.

Because the needle remains under the skin, irritation has been one of the major problems with this device. The most common resulting complication is infection. Obviously, if a needle is constantly present, there is a hole in the skin through which bacteria can enter. To minimize the possibility of infection, it is necessary to replace the tubing and the needle and to re-insert the needle in a new location every few days.

And for someone interested in sports—especially water sports—the external pump is definitely not a convenience.

Pump Implants

Another type of pump not yet as common as the external pump is one that is implanted in the abdominal wall. The surgery to insert this device is similar to that used for implanting a pacemaker. Since this device has no external features, nothing interferes with movement or provides an entrance to the body for infectious bacteria. The pump implant is therefore much more appealing than an external apparatus to active people.

Even though the initial implant does require minor surgery, the reservoir of the unit can be refilled and the batteries recharged without further surgery. Sensors operated by external electromagnetic units control the rate of flow, so the potential is there for longtime insulin delivery without frequent injections.

The insulin can be delivered directly to the portal blood vessels, the same vessels that naturally carry insulin from the pancreas to the liver. Or, it can be delivered into the abdominal space where it is rapidly absorbed into the portal blood vessels. As a result, the liver is the organ that gets most of the insulin first, which is what happens when the pancreas is functioning normally. Many people feel this is the ideal way to provide insulin, mimicking nature as closely as possible. However, the importance of the liver-first delivery is currently the subject of much debate. It certainly seems logical that this natural pathway would be best, yet we know that many diabetics do very well for years taking their insulin through injections under the skin. Some diabetologists theorize, however, that when the liver receives insulin directly, less insulin is required than when injection is the means of supply. Obviously, this economy could be a definite advantage to the diabetic.

Pancreas Transplants

The surgical technique with which surgeons have had the most experience involves removing about one half of the pancreas from a donor, based on current transplant procedures, and placing it in the recipient's body. To date, there have been just a few hundred of these transplants. Overall, relatively few of those patients have benefited.

In general, any transplant is major surgery—both risky and expensive. The major problem with transplanting an organ is the possibility of organ rejection. The recipient's body must accept not only the Islets of Langerhans, containing the beta cells that produce the insulin, but everything else in the pancreas as well, including the exocrine part, which produces digestive enzymes. The enzymes manufactured by a foreign pancreas can cause inflammation leading to pain, possible infection, and failure of the transplant.

Another potential risk, demonstrated recently in the case of a Type I diabetic who received a transplant from his identical twin, is that the same problem that destroyed the recipient's beta cells and originally brought on his diabetes may attack and selectively destroy the beta cells in the newly transplanted pancreas as well. (This appears to be less of a problem when the donor is not closely related to the recipient.)

Islet Transplants

You may well ask, if it is the exocrine cells of the pancreas that are causing the rejection, then why not just transplant the Islets of Langerhans? Researchers are, in fact, working on this procedure, and it does appear to have considerable promise.

There are, however, rejection problems with the islet transplants as well. Yet, major progress has been made in overcoming them. If researchers can overcome them completely, then the one remaining obstacle in making the procedure practical is the availability of enough islets from animal and human sources to help large numbers of people.

Researcher, Dr. Paul Lacy of Washington University in St. Louis has been able to take the islets from one species, i.e., mouse, and put them into another species, i.e., rat. That is a remarkable accomplishment and has spurred optimism that it may eventually be possible to make islet transplants from other animals to humans. The islets survived and functioned, curing diabetes without the need for major surgery or immune suppression drugs.

It is generally believed that Type I diabetics will benefit most from transplants. The Type I makes up only 10 percent of the diabetic population. At the present time, it is unclear but it appears unlikely that most Type II diabetics who do not require insulin will benefit from islet transplants.

Aldose Reductase Inhibitors

A great deal of work is currently underway to develop and test new drugs that will prevent the formation of sorbitol from glucose. These new compounds block (inhibit) the action of aldose reductase, the enzyme that converts glucose into sorbitol.

Because of their potential benefit, many different aldose reductase inhibitors are currently undergoing testing through several major pharmaceutical firms in the United States and overseas. These drugs are very effective in preventing vascular leakage, cataracts, and nerve damage in diabetic animals. They are now being tested in human diabetics to determine if nerve and eye damage from diabetes can be prevented and/or reversed. If

shown to be effective in these trials, they may be available in the near future for use by all diabetics.

This will not mean, however, that an insulin-requiring diabetic could do without insulin or that diet and exercise could be dispensed with. Nor would these drugs take the place of oral agents (discussed in Chapters 4 and 14). The appeal of these drugs is that they may be able to *prevent* many of the complications of diabetes without the need to *strictly* normalize blood glucose levels.

CHAPTER 18

Choosing a Doctor

Trying to find a family physician is not always an easy undertaking. Trying to choose a doctor who will treat diabetes with a goal toward normalizing blood sugar can be even more difficult. However, difficult does not mean impossible, and we hope that we can guide you here to successfully seek out someone who will help you.

We have given this particular problem a great deal of thought, finally concluding that the same advice given to patients who have to move to another city and find a new doctor would be applicable here, too.

The American Diabetes Association

Suppose, for example, your company transferred you from Missouri to Florida, and you asked for a reference for a new diabetologist. If we did not know any diabetologists there, we would advise you to contact the local chapter or the state affiliate of the American Diabetes Association, the American Medical Association, or the local medical society to seek names of diabetes specialists near you.

The Juvenile Diabetes Foundation

If you are the parent of a Type I diabetic, you might wish to contact the Juvenile Diabetes Foundation, which has lay chapters in many cities. Within the foundation, often there are support groups for parents of young diabetics. It is from those support groups that you might get the best leads regarding how the various diabetes experts are treating their patients. From the people within the support groups, you can find out how they feel about their respective physicians.

Everything we have discussed so far can, of course, be done right where you live. The channels just mentioned are ways in which to find knowledgeable medical help wherever you live.

Getting Leads

Getting leads, however, is only the beginning. For your own well-being, it is essential to expend some time and effort in the pursuit of proper care. To be sure you are getting a good doctor, you have to be reasonably well-informed and know the questions to ask (as you should by now, if you have read this book from the beginning).

As you know, we are convinced that normalization of blood glucose is currently the method that offers the most promise in preventing the complications of diabetes. Therefore, we urge you to see a physician who also is convinced of that. If the doctor is not convinced that normalization of blood sugar is important, then it is unlikely he or she will make the effort to educate patients to that end.

People often have difficulty communicating with their physicians when those doctors do not feel the need to explain what is causing problems. In the case of diabetes, it is important to ask the physician, point-blank, what he thinks it is that causes the complications. If he replies that the complications are genetic, it is unlikely that he will be as helpful to you in your efforts to normalize your blood sugars as would a physician who attributes complications to poor blood sugar control. Also ask about diet and exercise. Be sure the physician will spend the time himself or have an educator who will help you practice good nutrition.

If the physician tells you that preventing complications is in "some way" related to the control of blood glucose levels, find out his or her attitude regarding normalization of these levels. If he is going to be able to help you, he must be knowledgeable about different methods of insulin treatment and self glucose monitoring. He must be interested in multiple injections or a pump if you are an insulin-dependent diabetic. If he is not using those techniques for at least some of his patients, then it is unlikely that he will be able to provide you with the best possible help.

Not All "Experts" Are Experts

As a word of caution, do not accept the designation of a physician as a diabetologist or as a diabetes expert at face value. There are diabetes experts who know a lot about the causes and problems of diabetes but do not know enough about practical diabetes management to help effectively. If you find someone good, but with a practice so busy that the doctor cannot take you as a patient, ask that physician or a member of the staff to recommend another physician. The good ones know about the other good ones.

You have the right and the responsibility to find a doctor who will provide the care, support, advice, and information you want. *You,* however good the doctor is, will still have to exercise the responsibility to direct your own life every day, through diet, exercise, and medication to achieve the good control you need. It is a big assignment, but it is achievable with the proper knowledge, motivation, and medical help.

Best wishes as you set forth on the road to good control—and a healthier, longer life.

Appendix A

Resources

American Association of Diabetes Educators
500 N. Michigan Ave.
Suite 1400
Chicago, Ill. 60611

American Diabetes Association
1660 Duke Street, P.O. Box 25757
Alexandria, Va. 22314

American Dietetic Association
430 North Michigan Avenue
Chicago, Ill. 60611

Joslin Diabetes Clinic
One Joslin Place
Boston, Mass. 02215

Juvenile Diabetes Foundation
23 East 26th Street
New York, N.Y. 10010

Kilo Diabetes & Vascular Research Foundation
1227 Fern Ridge Parkway
Suite 100
St. Louis, Mo. 63141

Suggested Reading and References

American Diabetes Association. *Guide to Good Living*. ADA Inc., National Service Center, 1660 Duke Street, P.O. Box 25757, Alexandria, Va. 22314.

Anderson, J.W. *Diabetes: A Practical New Guide to Healthy Living.* Featuring the HCF Diet Program (New York: Arco Publishing Inc., 1981).

Bierman, J. and Toohey, B. *The Diabetes Question and Answer Book.* (Sherbourne Press, 1976).

Bierman, J. and Toohey, B. *The Diabetic's Book, All Your Questions Answered.* (Los Angeles: J.P. Tarcher Inc., 1981).

Bierman, J. and Toohey, B. *The Diabetic's Total Health Book.* (Los Angeles: J.P. Tarcher Inc., 1980).

Bierman, J. and Toohey, B. *The Diabetic's Sports and Exercise Book.* (Philadelphia: J.B. Lippincott, 1977).

Danowski, T.S. *Diabetes as a Way of Life.* (New York: Coward-McCann, 1974).

Jorgensen, C.D. and Lewis, J.E. *The ABCs of Diabetes.* (New York: Crown, 1979).

Kilo, C. *Educating the Diabetic Patient.* (New York: Science and Medicine, 1982).

Kilo, C. and Dudley, J. *Self Blood Glucose Monitoring, For the Person with Diabetes Mellitus.* (Chicago: American Association of Diabetes Educators, 1984).

Kivelowitz, T. *Diabetes.* (Englewood Cliffs, N.J.: Prentice-Hall, 1981).

Krall, L., and Beaser, R. *Joslin Diabetes Manual,* 12th ed. (Philadelphia: Lea & Febiger, 1988).

Laufer, L.J. and Kadison, H. *Diabetes Explained: A Layman's Guide.* (New York: E.P. Dutton, 1976).

Lodewick, P. *A Diabetic Doctor Looks at Diabetes, His and Yours.* (Cambridge, Mass.: RMI Corporation, 1982).

A Medicine in the Public Interest Publication. *Learning to Live with Diabetes.* 1984. Write to Suite 304, 65 Franklin Street, Boston, Mass. 02110.

Milchovich, S., Dunn, B.L., Snydergaard, T., and Rettinger, H.I. *Diabetes Mellitus . . . What's It All About?* Anaheim Memorial Hospital, California Community Health Education Center, Anaheim, 1982.

Mirsky, S. and Heilman, J.R. *Diabetes: Controlling It the Easy Way.* (New York: Random House, 1981).

Moore, Michael V., ed. *Learning to Live Well with Diabetes.* (Minneapolis, Mn.: International Diabetes Center, 1985).

Peterson, C.M. *Take Charge of Your Diabetes: A New Approach to Self-Management.* Self-published, 1979. (Order through P.O. Box 802, South Bend, Ind.).

Pray, L.M. and Evans, R. *Journey of a Diabetic.* (New York: Simon & Schuster, 1983).

Reeves-Ellington, ed. *Blood Glucose Monitoring: For the Phases of Your Life.* (New York: Health Education Technologies, 1986).

Sims, D.F. *Diabetes: Reach for Health and Freedom.* (St. Louis: C.V. Mosby Co., 1984).

The National Diabetes Information Clearing House. *The Diabetes Dictionary.* Box NDIC, Bethesda, Maryland 20205.

Appendix C

Cookbooks for Diabetics

American Diabetes Association and the American Dietetic Association. *Family Cookbook.* Vols. I (1980) and II (1984), (Englewood Cliffs, N.J.: Prentice-Hall, Inc.).

American Diabetes Association and the American Dietetic Association. *Exchange Lists for Meal Planning.* 1976. Write to American Diabetes Association, 1660 Duke Street, P.O. Box 25757, Alexandria, Va. 22513.

Franz, M. *Exchanges for All Occasions.* Meeting the Challenge of Diabetes, 1983. Write to Park Nicollet Medical Foundation, 4959 Excelsior Boulevard, Minneapolis, Minn. 55416.

Jones, J. *More Calculated Cooking.* (San Francisco: 101 Productions, 1981).

Majors, J. *Sugar Free . . . That's Me!* (New York: Ballantine Books, 1980).

Middleton, K. and Hess, M.A. *The Art of Cooking for the Diabetic.* (New York: Signet Books, 1979).

Moe, J., Rubin, K., and Abrams, S. *The No Sugar Delicious Dessert Cookbook.* (Berkeley, Ca.: Celestial Arts, 1984).

Note: Cookbooks and Suggested Reading and References are intended to be neither complete nor recommended lists. Rather they include the publications the authors are most familiar with. A complete list of publications, cookbooks, etc. for people with diabetes can be obtained from the:

U.S. Department of Health and Human Services
National Diabetes Information Clearing House
Box NDIC
Bethesda, Md. 20892
301-468-2162

Index

Acromegaly, 30
Adrenal corticosteroids, 170
Adrenal glands, 24
Adrenaline, 66, 169–171
Adult-onset diabetes, *See* Type II diabetes
"Age peaks," 21–22
Aging, metabolism and, 65–66
Alcohol:
  excess glucose and, 100
  liver and, 142
  metabolism and, 49–50
Aldose reductase inhibitors, 180
Alpha cells, 7, 9, 10, 61, 135, 136
American Association of Diabetes Educators, (AADE), 122, 129, 187
American Diabetes Association, 114, 183, 187, 188, 191
American Dietetic Association, 187, 191
American Medical Association, 114
Amino acids:
  glucose and, 31, 78, 135
  insulin and, 6
  liver and, 13, 78
Aneurysms, 51
Anger, 169, 171, 172
Angina, 48
Antigens, 57, 58, 61, 91
Aorta, 44
Appetite, regulators of, 64
Arteries, *See* Blood vessels
Athletes, 35, 142–145

Beta cells, 7, 9–11, 94, 135, 136
  antibodies to, 20
  antigens, 61
  destruction: "honeymoon" stage, 22
  genes, 58
  insulin "factory," 93
  insulin production: fat/thin persons, 27–28
  pancreatitis, 31
  Type II diabetics, 25
  viral infections, 21
Biofeedback, 13, 174
Bladder infections, 72
Blindness, 98, 51
Blood pressure, High, 44
Blood sugar/glucose level:
  controlled; good feeling, 23
  controversy on value of control, 114
  high; danger, 99–101
  monitoring, 106
  "normal," 24
  normalization of, 131–148
  scar tissue and, 44
  self-monitoring, 128, 129, 138–140, 144, 170
  tests, 138
  See also Glucose; Insulin; Treatment
Blood vessels:
  aneurysms in capillaries, 51
  arteries, capillaries, veins, 44
  coronary artery (figure), 47
  elasticity, 43
  leaky, 44–45
  scar tissue; closing, 47
  thigh muscle capillary (figure), 105
Borderline diabetes, 24

Brain:
  cell regeneration, 43
  cells, 15, 136
  damage, 137
  energy use, 14
  glucose needs of, 136, 137
  operation, 136–137
  transient impairment, 48

Calories:
  burnt by exercise (table), 143
  estimating needs, 131–132
  ideal body weight and, 132
  meal/snack plan (1825 calories), 162–164
  stress and, 66–67
  See also Food(s)
Capillaries, *See* Blood vessels
Carbohydrates:
  energy, 14
  frequency of diabetes and, 60
  metabolism of, 7
  water-soluble, 15
Cardiovascular disease, 98, 104, 107
Cardiovascular system:
  strengths and weaknesses, 42–47
  symptoms of damage, 48
Cataracts, 100
Cells:
  glucose-burning, 15
  obesity: resistant to insulin, 27–28
  scar tissue and, 43
Childbearing, 71, 77
Cholesterol:
  content of various foods (table), 164–167
  hazard, 41
  high insulin levels and, 99
  leaky blood vessels, 44, 45
  lipoproteins, 6
  scarring process and, 44, 47
Cigarette smoking, 44, 46, 74, 79, 148
Circulation (blood), 48
Claudication, 48
Coma, 17, 18, 20, 136, 137
Concentration, and stress, 173
Control, 4, 5, 95, 140
Cookbooks, 191–192
Coping, 4
Coxsackie B-4, 60
C-peptide, 93–94
Cures, dangerous hopes, 175
Cushing's disease, 30
Cystic fibrosis, 31

Death, diabetes as factor in; statistics, 54–55
Depression, 89, 123
Diabetes:
  cases, 19–20
  cause: lack of insulin, 5–6, 99
  complications, 54, 97–108
  definition, 4
  the diabetes educator, *See* Education
  genes in Types I and II differ, 57
  groups, 4, 11. *See also* Type I, Type II
  insulin, *See* Insulin
  living a healthier life, 33–39
  mistaken notions about, 3
  patients, difficult to control, 104, 106

potential diabetics, 31–32
signs, first, 16–18
treatment, *See* Treatment
Diet:
active, healthy living, 33
adaptation to habits, 132–134
food, 140–144
normalization of glucose levels, 131
personalized, 37
planning, 149–167
proportions of food groups, 60
variety not sacrificed, 140–143
See also Calories; Fasting; Food(s); Meals
Digestion, 12
Doctor(s), choosing, 183–185
"Down regulation," 28

Eating:
counseling the diabetic, 122–123
developing better habits, 68–69
prudence in, 59–60
times related to injections, 133
See also Overeating
Education:
the diabetes educator, 121–129
essential in treatment, 119–129
gradual approach, 124
the juvenile diabetic, 125–127
survival skills, 124–125
Ejaculation, 82
Emotions, 5, 123, 172
Endocrine pancreas, 7
Energy:
oxygen and, 14
short-term needs, 14
storage: fat, 14
Environment, 58–61
Epinephrine, *See* Adrenaline
Erection, 81
Exercise, 142
beneficial effects, 36
compensating for (diet), 133, 143–145
importance, 38, 133, 142–145
right kind of, 36–37
stress and, 173
Exocrine pancreas, 9
"Experts," 185
Eye examinations, 51

Fasting:
blood sugar level, 24
body reaction to, 67
long-term; detrimental, 38
salt-to-water imbalance, 67
Fat cells, 64, 68
Fatty acids (fats):
cells, 15
energy, storage of, 14
insulin and, 6
ketones, 17
lipoproteins, 45
See also Food(s)
Fear, 169
Fetus:
differentiation process, 74
high blood sugar, 74
lung maturation, 75
normal development, 73–74
one-dose-a-day insulin, 77, 134
Fiber (foods), 153, 161
Flu, 20, 21

Food(s), 149–167
See also Calories; Eating; Meals
Foot care, 50

Gangrene, 47, 50
Genes, 53, 57, 97
Genetics, 53, 56
Gestational diabetes, 76
Glucagon, 7, 135, 137
Glucocorticoids, 30–31
Glucose:
cells burning sugar, 15
a carbohydrate, 14
excess, 45, 99–101
fasting and, 67
high level of, in bloodstream, 9, 10, 12, 16
insulin and, 6, 29
nerve damage, 46
self blood glucose monitor, 78, 138–140, 147
See also Blood sugar/glucose level
Glucose tolerance tests, 17(note)
Glycogen, 12, 13, 38
Glycohemoglobin measurement, 106, 127
Glycosylation, 46, 100–101
Grieving, 3, 123
Guilt, and stress, 172, 173

Healing, 48
Heart, cell regeneration in, 43
Heart attack, 47, 110
Heart disease, 78–79, 113
Hemochromatosis, 31
Heredity:
diabetic complications, 54, 104
obesity and, 53
Siperstein's findings and, 103
Type II diabetes, 56
High blood sugar, *See* Blood sugar/glucose level; Hyperglycemia
"Honeymoon" stage, 22
Hormones, 13, 107, 135
Hunger, 64
Hyperglycemia:
causes, 30
potential diabetics, 32
scarring process and, 44
serious nature of, 4
sorbitol, 45–46
See also Blood sugar/glucose level
Hyperthyroidism, 65
Hypoglycemia:
insulin shock, 136
newborn babies, 74, 77
oral agents and, 146
Hypothalamus, 64
Hypothyroidism, 65

Immune response, 57–58
Implants–pump, 178
Impotence, 72–73
organic disturbances, 83
permanent, 82
psychological causes, 83
Infants, 74, 75, 77, 78
Infections:
glucocorticoids, 31
vaginal and urinary tract, 23, 72
virus theory, 21
Influenza, 20, 21
Insulin:
binding failure, 29
chemical composition, 93
complications related to lack, 99

deficiency; metabolism, 11
dosage amount, 134–138
extraction and preparation of, 91
factors related to need, 35
function utilizing food, 6, 15
glucose moved through cells by, 15
injections: times related to eatng, 132–133
lack: root cause of diabetes, 5–6
need dictated by insufficiency, 34
one-dose-a-day, 77, 94, 134
pregnancy, 74–78
production: fat/thin persons, 27
pro-insulin, 93
purification process, 92
receptors on fat cells, 68
regular schedule, 148
storage, 93
synthesized, 92
who must take? 34–35
See also Diabetes
Insulin pumps, 176–177
Insulin resistance, 11, 28
failure to bind to receptors (figure), 29
reduction in receptors, 68
women, 71
Insulin shock, 133–138
Iron, 31, 153
Islets of Langerhans, 7, 94, 135, 179
diagram, 9, 10
insulin (origin of the word), 89
transplants, 179–180

Juvenile Diabetes Foundation, 184, 187
Juvenile diabetics, 125–127
Juvenile-onset diabetes,
See Type I diabetes
Ketoacidosis, 17, 76, 77, 78, 94, 97, 134–135
Ketones, 17, 78
Kidneys, 48
Kilo, C., 109, 115, 189
Kilo Diabetes & Vascular Research
Foundation, 102, 187

Langerhans, Paul, 7, 89.
See also Islets of Langerhans
Lipoproteins, 6, 45
Liver:
alcohol and, 142
amino acids, 13, 78
biofeedback system, 13
diagram, 13
glucose production; not eating, 78, 133–134
metabolism and insulin deficiency, 11, 12
oral agents, 146
Lung maturation (fetus), 75
Lung tissue, renewal of, 47

Malpractice suits, 110
Maturity-onset diabetes,
See Type II diabetes
Meals, 24, 38, 95, 148, 149
See also Diet; Food(s)
Medication, *See* Insulin; Oral agents
Meditation, 174
Men:
diabetics, 81–85
impotence, 73, 81, 82
penile implant, 81, 83–85
reproductive concerns, 85
Metabolism:
aging and, 65–66
alcohol and, 49–50
efficiency differences, 15
evolution of, 14–15
insulin deficiency, 11
mice and humans, 53
rate of, 15
regulators of, 64
survival depends on, 12
utilization, 12
Mice:
genetic similarity to humans, 53
obesity, 55
susceptibility to diabetes, 56
virus inoculation, 60
Miscarriage, 74
Monoject Insulin Reaction Gel, 138, 143
Morning sickness, 77–78
Motivation, 128
Muscles:
atrophy, 52
cells, 15
fasting and, 38
liver uses amino acids from, 13
Myo-inositol, 45

National Diabetes Information Clearing
House, 190, 192
Needles, new, 176
Nerves:
alcohol and, 49–50
"bad nerves," 49–50
damage, 45, 46, 100
fibers; insulation, 49
glucose; permeability, 49
Neuropathy, 49, 50, 82, 98
Nobel Prize, 90
Noncompliance, 112
Normalization, vi
See also Blood sugar/glucose level

Obesity:
cause, 60
fat cells get bigger, 16
heredity and, 53
how we get fat, 63
hypothalamus damage, 64–65
insulin producing, 27
predisposition, 55–57
women, 71
Oral agents:
alternative to insulin treatment, 35
different objectives, 146
during pregnancy, 77
educating the patient, 121
monitoring effectiveness of, 147
potentially dangerous, 147
research on, 110
Type II diabetes, 146
unresponsiveness to, 147
Orgasm, 73
Overeating, 29, 56, 57, 59, 61
Overweight, 23, 24, 25, 36, 99, 146
Oxygen, 14

Pancreas:
anatomy (figure), 8
insulin production 28–29
insulin reserve in, 56
potential diabetics, 31–32
role of, 7–11
strain: insulin resistance, 68
transplants, 179
Type II diabetics, 26, 27
Pancreatitis, 31
Parents, 126

Penile implant, 81, 83–85
Penis, 73, 82
Phenformin, 110, 113–114
Physicans, choosing a doctor, 183–185
Pituitary gland, 30, 65
Poisons, causing diabetes, 61
Potassium, 136, 153, 160, 161
Pregnancy, 73–78
  insulin: extra demand for, 75–77
  oral agents not approved, 77
  risk of congenital malformation, 73
  susceptibility of offspring, 78
  temporary diabetes during, 76–78
  Types I/II diabetics, 77
  underdeveloped big babies, 75
  See also Fetus
Pro-insulin, 93
Prostheses, 83
Proteins, 60
Pumps, 176–178

Rejection, 91
Relaxation, 173
Renal failure, 48
Renal threshold, 16, 139, 140
Research:
  computers in, 111–112
  counter-findings (to Siperstein), 103–104
  first effective treatment, 90
  injury to nerves and vessels, 106
  long learning process, 89
  noncompliance of patients, 112
  on prevention of complications, 109
  University Group Diabetes Program (UGDP), 109
Retina, 51

Scar tissue:
  blood vessels, 47
  cell regeneration and, 43
  cholesterol, 44
  eye problems, 51
  reversal, 46–47
Schwann cells, 49, 50
Seasonal trends, 20–21
Secondary diabetes, 30–31
Sexual function, effect of diabetes on, 72–73
Siperstein, Marvin, 101–104, 108
Sodium, 136
Sorbitol, 45–46, 49, 100, 180
Sports, 37, 142–145
Steroid treatment, 31
Stress:
  adrenaline and, 169–171
  alleviating, 169–174
  blood sugar level, 24
  calories burnt up in, 66–67
  cause, 172
  controlling, 171–174
  exercise and, 173
  glucocorticoids, 31
  positive focus, 173
  signs of, 171
"Strip test," 17
Stroke, 47, 48
Sugar, refined, 60

Thiamin, 153
Thin persons, 27, 63
Thyroid gland, 65
Thyroxine, 65
Tolbutamide, 110, 113–114
Transient ischemic attacks (TIA's), 48
Transplants, 91, 179–180
Treatment:
  attitude: dangerous hopes, 175
  blood glucose level; normalization, 119
  catastrophic problems from improper treatment, 41–42
  development of new drugs, 114(note)
  early; severity, 119
  education essential in, 119–129
  first effective treatment (1921), 90
  proper; healthy, active living, 33
  self blood glucose monitoring, 78, 134, 138
  Siperstein's findings and, 103
Tumors, 30, 31
Twins, identical, 57
Type I (insulin-dependent) diabetes:
  age peaks, 21–22
  antibodies to beta cells, 20
  beta cells in, 11, 94
  case: sudden onset, rapid progression, 19–20
  characteristics, 22–23
  definition, 4
  genetic susceptibility, 21
  "honeymoon" stage, 22
  immune response and, 57–58
  influenza and, 20, 21
  insulin needed in, 34–35; *See also* Insulin
  new technology for management, 176–181
  onset of symptoms, 103
  prediction of high risk, 58
  seasonal trend of onset, 20–21
  susceptibility to, 56–57
  urine sugar, 20
  weight loss, 20
Type II (non-insulin-dependent) diabetes:
  beta cells in, 11, 25
  definition, 4
  degrees; diagnosis, 24
  development (gradual), 23
  hereditary factors, 56
  infections, 23
  insulin needed in, 34–35; *See also* Insulin
  oral agents, 146
  Siperstein's experiment, 102
  susceptibility to, 55–56
  oral agents (medication), 35
  symptoms, 23
  treatment effectiveness (research), 109
  typical victims, 23, 25, 46

United States Supreme Court, 111
University Group Diabetes Program (UGDP), 109
Urinalysis, 16–17
Urinary tract infections, 23, 72
Urine sugar:
  checking/testing, 78, 134, 139–140, 147
  infections in women, 72
  sign of diabetes, 16, 20

Vaginal tract infections, 23, 72
Vascular system, *See* Cardiovascular system
Viruses, as cause of diabetes, 60–61
Vitamins, 160, 161

Weight:
  frequency of diabetes related to, 59
  ideal, 24–25, 68, 131–132
  loss, 20
  See also Overweight; Obesity
Williamson, Joseph R., 109, 189
Women, 71–79